THE COMMON SYMPTOM GUIDE

THE COMMON SYMPTOM GUIDE

A guide to the evaluation of 100
common adult and pediatric symptoms

John Wasson, M.D.
Robert Wood Johnson Clinical Scholar
Stanford Medical School

B. Timothy Walsh, M.D.
Resident in Psychiatry
Albert Einstein College of Medicine

Richard Tompkins, M.D.
Assistant Professor of Medicine
Dartmouth Medical School;
Director, Dartmouth Promis Laboratory

Harold Sox, Jr., M.D.
Assistant Professor of Medicine
Stanford Medical School;
Director, Palo Alto Veteran's Hospital Ambulatory Care Project

McGraw-Hill Book Company

A Blakiston Publication

**New York   St. Louis   San Francisco   Auckland   Düsseldorf
Johannesburg   Kuala Lumpur   London   Mexico   Montreal
New Delhi   Panama   Paris   São Paulo   Singapore   Sydney
Tokyo   Toronto**

Notice

Medicine is an ever-changing science. As new research and clinical experience broaden our knowledge, changes in treatment and drug therapy are required. The editors and the publisher of this work have made every effort to ensure that the drug dosage schedules herein are accurate and in accord with the standards accepted at the time of publication. The reader is advised, however, to check the product information sheet included in the package of each drug he plans to administer to be certain that changes have not been made in the recommended dose or in the contraindications for administration. This recommendation is of particular importance in regard to new or infrequently used drugs.

Library of Congress Cataloging in Publication Data
Main entry under title:

The Common symptom guide.

"A Blakiston publication."
1. Semiology. 2. Diagnosis. I. Wasson, John.
[DNLM: 1. Diagnosis, Differential. 2. Medicine.
3. Pediatrics. WB141 C734]
RC69.C76   616.07'2   75-5757
ISBN 0-07-068435-9

THE COMMON SYMPTOM GUIDE

4567891011I2 MUMU 9

IN MEMORY OF

David B. Kaner, M.D.
Margaret Little Long

> "Unique human beings, loved
> and respected by all who
> knew them".

The Common Symptom Guide is intended for the student of clinical medicine who needs to know what historical data and physical examination are relevant to a patient's symptoms. Most standard medical textbooks deal in depth with disease but provide relatively little help in evaluating symptoms. The Common Symptom Guide deals in depth with symptom evaluation. It provides a listing of pertinent questions, physical findings, and differential diagnosis for each of one hundred common adult and pediatric symptoms. It is intended to provide the busy practitioner, physician's assistant, nurse or medical student with an overview of the causes of the symptoms and the information to distinguish between them.

There is little experimental evidence about what clinical data are really necessary to evaluate a symptom correctly. Since we feel that the history and physical examination are a relatively inexpensive and risk-free part of health care, this edition of the Guide is probably more complete than may actually be required in practice. On the other hand, since the Guide is directed toward the symptoms caused by relatively common diseases, the subspecialist may find it incomplete. The user of the Common Symptom Guide should be aware of its potential inadequacies and help the authors to remedy them in future editions.

The information found in the Guide comes principally from the following textbooks:

Textbook of Pediatrics, Edited by: Waldo I. Nelson, Victor Vaughan, R. James McKay, 10th Edition, W.B. Saunders Company, Philadelphia, 1975.

Common Symptoms of Diseases of Children, R.S. Illingworth, R.A. Davis Company, Philadelphia, 1969.

Principles of Surgery, Seymour I. Schwartz, Editor and Chief, McGraw Hill Book Company, New York, 1974.

Family Practice, Edited by: Howard F. Conn, Robert E. Rakel and Thomas W. Johnson, W.B. Saunders Company, Philadelphia. 1973.

The Principles and Practice of Medicine, Edited by: A. McGehee Harvey, Richard J. Johns, Albert H. Owens, Jr., Richard S. Ross, Eighteenth Edition, Appleton-Century-Crofts, Merideth Corporation, New York, 1972.

Harrison's Principles of Internal Medicine, Edited by: Maxwell Wintrobe, George W. Thorne, Raymond D. Adams, Eugene Braunwald, Kurt J. Isselbacher, Robert G. Petersdorf, Seventh Edition, McGraw Hill Book Company, New York, 1974.

When possible, specific page references to <u>Harrison's Principles of Internal Medicine</u> are provided to direct the reader to more comprehensive discussion, since this book does not describe laboratory methods of evaluation or therapy.

This book is intended to be used at the bedside or in the office. The inexperienced student of health care should use the <u>Guide</u> as a reminder of what to do and ask. More experienced health care personnel can use the <u>Guide</u> as a standard of personal performance, modifying it in accordance with their clinical needs.

> John Wasson, M.D.
> B. Timothy Walsh, M.D.
> Richard Tompkins, M.D.
> Harold Sox, Jr., M.D.
>
> January 1975.

We wish to express our appreciation to the following special contributors who have reviewed the manuscript.

James F. Fries, M.D. (Rheumatology)
   Stanford University School of Medicine

Michael F. Marmor, M.D. (Opthalmology)
   Stanford University School of Medicine

Robert B. Pantell, M.D. (Pediatrics)
   Stanford University School of Medicine

George Perlstein, M.D. (Neurology)
   Palo Alto Medical Clinic

Robert Porter, M.D. (Orthopedic Surgery)
   Dartmouth Hitchcock Medical Center

Carl Sadowsky, M.D. (Neurology)
   Dartmouth Hitchcock Medical Center

Edward R. Silverblatt, M.D. (Gastroenterology)
   Stanford University School of Medicine

Stephen Spencer, M.D. (Dermatology)
   Dartmouth Hitchcock Medical Center

We also wish to express our gratitude to the nurses, medical students, physician's assistants, and physicians whose criticism has been so valuable. We are particularly indebted to Janet Brandsma, Beverly Kusler, Sony Lipton and Peggy Goldman for their assistance in preparing the manuscript.

Partial support for this work was provided by the National Fund for Medical Education Grant #57/71 to Dartmouth Medical School and by the Robert Wood Johnson Foundation through the Stanford University Clinical Scholars Program.

THE INDEX

The <u>Common Symptom Guide</u> specifies what to ask and what parts of the physical examination to perform for the evaluation of each of one hundred symptoms. Each of these symptoms is CAPITALIZED in the Index and appear in the text in alphabetical order.

Many other symptoms are listed in the Index. The evaluation of these non-capitalized symptoms is covered under the CAPITALIZED symptom which is listed nearby in the Index. Thus, for the patient complaining of "weakness", the user will find reference to DEPRESSION, LETHARGY and MUSCLE WEAKNESS listed adjacent to "weakness" in the Index. The user can turn to the Data Base page whose title best describes the patient's complaint.

Potentially life threatening symptoms are identified in the Index by asterisks (e.g. CHEST PAIN*).

THE MEDICATIONS SECTION

Patients may not remember the names of medications that have been prescribed for them. The user of the <u>GUIDE</u> may aid a patient in recalling these medications by referring to the Medications Section and naming some of the common drugs prescribed for the patient's problem. Thus, if the patient is taking a "blue blood pressure pill", the mention of "hydralazine" found under "blood pressure" in the Medications Section may make positive identification possible. The physical description of the medication may be a further aid to identification.

THE DIRECTED DATA BASE SECTION

A. For every symptom the user of the <u>Common Symptom Guide</u> must always ask the following descriptors (reproduced on the inside front cover).

1. The patient's age.
2. The mode of onset of a symptom:
   a. Description of events coincident with onset.
   b. Whether there have been similar episodes in the past.
   c. Whether the onset was gradual or sudden.
   d. The total duration of the symptom.

3. The location of the symptom (if applicable). The location should be anatomically precise.
4. The character of the symptom (e.g. dull, sharp or burning pain).
5. The radiation of the symptom (if applicable). Radiation of the symptom (the pattern of spread) is most often applicable to a patient's description of pain or an abnormal sensation.
6. Precipitating or aggravating factors.
7. Relieving or ameliorating factors.
8. Past treatment or evaluation of the symptom.
    a. When, where, and by whom?
    b. What studies were performed in the past and what were the results? (i.e. blood studies, x-rays, etc).
    c. Results of past treatment.
    d. Past diagnosis.
9. Course of the symptom (getting worse, getting better).
10. Effect of the symptom on normal daily activities.

B. Specific information to be obtained for each symptom is presented on the Data Base page using the following format.

HISTORY

Descriptors:

General Descriptors:
Onset:
Location:
Character:
Radiation:
Aggravating factors:
Relieving factors:
Past treatment or evaluation:

Specific descriptors listed here will be those considered particularly important for the evaluation of the symptom. The user will always be expected to ask the general descriptors listed in Section A above and reproduced on the inside front cover.

Associated Symptoms:

Medical History:

Medications:

Family History:

Environmental History:

False Positive Considerations:

Specific information will be requested which is considered important for the evaluation of the symptom.

PHYSICAL EXAMINATION

This section will specify the parts of the physical examination that are considered necessary to evaluate the symptom.

Data necessary for pediatric evaluation is generally identified as such and incorporated into the Data Base pages except where this approach seems inappropriate. Thus, for example, ABDOMINAL PAIN has a section for both adults and children.

THE GLOSSARY

A glossary of terms used in the HISTORY section of the Data Base pages is included at the end of the Common Symptom Guide.

PSYCHOLOGICAL CONSIDERATIONS:

The risk of the Common Symptom Guide

A correct problem solving strategy is based on correctly defining the problem. The symptom that a patient describes may not be the only reason that medical attention was sought. In fact, it may be a pretext to gain the privacy of a physician's office to disclose concerns of a very personal nature that would be embarrassing to disclose in a crowded waiting room. Health care workers who base their evaluation on the narrowest possible grounds, the patient's complaint, may take needless diagnostic or therapeutic measures because they have failed to identify the real problem.

The Guide frequently identifies those symptoms which are likely to have significant emotional components. Nevertheless, it remains the duty of those using this book to be sensitive to the unspoken words, gestures, and multiple ill-defined complaints which may indicate the patient's desire for emotional evaluation and support.

THE GENERAL INDEX

SYMPTOM

abdominal pain	ABDOMINAL PAIN* BLOOD IN STOOL* ULCER, GASTRIC VOMITING BLOOD*
abortion	ABORTION* VAGINAL BLEEDING PROBLEMS
abrasion-laceration	ABRASION-LACERATION TRAUMA*
abscess	ABSCESS LUMP-LYMPHADENOPATHY ULCERS-LEG
accident	ABRASION-LACERATION* HEAD INJURY* TRAUMA*
aches	ABDOMINAL PAIN* BACK PAIN CHEST PAIN* DEPRESSION EAR PROBLEMS FACIAL PAIN HEADACHE JOINT-EXTREMITY PAIN NECK PAIN UPPER RESPIRATORY INFECTION
acne	ADOLESCENT-PUBERTY PROBLEMS SKIN PROBLEMS
adolescent-puberty problems	ADOLESCENT-PUBERTY PROBLEMS
alcoholism	ALCOHOLISM
allergies	ALLERGIES ASTHMA SKIN PROBLEMS
amblyopia	DOUBLE VISION EYE PROBLEMS
amenorrhea	VAGINAL BLEEDING PROBLEMS
anemia	ANEMIA LETHARGY
angina	ANGINA* CHEST PAIN*
ankle injury	ABRASION-LACERATION* FOOT-ANKLE PROBLEMS
anorexia	ANOREXIA DEPRESSION SMALL BABY (PEDIATRIC)
anus problems	ANUS PROBLEMS BLOOD IN STOOL*
anxiety	DEPRESSION

* Potentially life threatening symptom

aphasia	TALKING TROUBLE
appendix	ABDOMINAL PAIN*
appetite	ANOREXIA EXCESSIVE EATING
arm pain	ANGINA* CHEST PAIN* HAND-WRIST-ARM PAIN JOINT-EXTREMITY PAIN TRAUMA*
arrhythmia	PALPITATIONS
arthritis	JOINT-EXTREMITY PAIN
asthma	ALLERGIES ASTHMA BREATHING TROUBLE*
ataxia	GAIT-COORDINATION PROBLEMS
back pain	ABDOMINAL PAIN* BACK PAIN URINE TROUBLE
bad breath	MOUTH TROUBLE
balance	GAIT-COORDINATION PROBLEMS
baldness	HAIR CHANGE
beaten up	HEAD INJURY* TRAUMA*
bed wetting	BED WETTING
behavior-irritability	BEHAVIOR-IRRITABILITY (PEDIATRIC) CONFUSION* HYPERACTIVITY (PEDIATRIC)
belching	INDIGESTION
birth control	BIRTH CONTROL
bitten, insect	ALLERGIES
bitten - other	ABRASION-LACERATION*

* Potentially life threatening symptom

SYMPTOM

black out	BLACK OUT* CONVULSION* DIZZY-VERTIGO UNCONSCIOUS*
black stools	BLOOD IN STOOLS*
bladder trouble	DARK URINE URINE TROUBLE
bleeding	(specify site) BRUISING-BLEEDING TENDENCY*
bloating	ABDOMINAL PAIN* INDIGESTION SWELLING
blood, coughing up	COUGHING BLOOD VOMITING BLOOD*
blood in stools	BLOOD IN STOOLS*
blood in urine	DARK URINE
blood in vomit	VOMITING BLOOD*
blood pressure	HYPERTENSION
bloody nose	NOSE-SINUS PROBLEMS
blue color skin	BREATHING TROUBLE* CYANOSIS*
blurred vision	DOUBLE VISION EYE PROBLEMS
boil	ABSCESS LUMP-LYMPHADENOPATHY ULCER, LEG
bowel problems	ABDOMINAL PAIN* ANUS PROBLEMS BLOOD IN STOOL* CONSTIPATION DIARRHEA
breast problems	BREAST PROBLEMS
breathing trouble	BREATHING TROUBLE* CHEST PAIN* COUGH
bronchitis	ASTHMA BREATHING TROUBLE* COUGH
bruising-bleeding tendency	BRUISING-BLEEDING TENDENCY*
bump	HEAD INJURY* LUMP-LYMPHADENOPATHY TRAUMA*

* Potentially life threatening symptom

bunion	FOOT-ANKLE PROBLEM
burn	BURN*
burning urination	URINE TROUBLE
burping	INDIGESTION
bursitis	JOINT-EXTREMITY PAIN
buzzing in ear	DIZZY-VERTIGO EAR PROBLEMS
calf pain	JOINT-EXTREMITY PAIN
cancer	ANOREXIA BLOOD IN STOOL* COUGHING BLOOD JAUNDICE* LUMP-LYMPHADENOPATHY WEIGHT LOSS
cataract	EYE PROBLEMS
change of life	DEPRESSION VAGINAL BLEEDING PROBLEMS
change in feeding	ANOREXIA BEHAVIOR-IRRITABILITY
chest pain	ANGINA* BREATHING TROUBLE* CHEST PAIN*
chills	FEVER*
choking	BREATHING TROUBLE* DIFFICULTY SWALLOWING
cirrhosis	ALCOHOLISM JAUNDICE*
clap	VD
claudication	JOINT-EXTREMITY PAIN
clumsiness	GAIT-COORDINATION
cold	COUGH UPPER RESPIRATORY INFECTION
cold sore	MOUTH TROUBLE

* Potentially life threatening symptom

SYMPTOM

colic (Pediatric)	ABDOMINAL PAIN*
colitis	ABDOMINAL PAIN* DIARRHEA
coma	CONVULSIONS* HEAD TRAUMA* OVERDOSE* UNCONSCIOUS*
confusion	CONFUSION* HEAD TRAUMA*
conjunctivitis	EYE PROBLEMS
congestion	COUGH NOSE-SINUS TROUBLE
constipation	CONSTIPATION
contraception	BIRTH CONTROL
convulsions	CONVULSIONS* TWITCHING
coordination problems	GAIT-COORDINATION
coronary	CHEST PAIN*
cough	COUGH
coughing blood	COUGHING BLOOD VOMITING BLOOD*
cramps-menstrual	ABDOMINAL PAIN* CRAMPS-MENSTRUAL
cramps-muscular	JOINT-EXTREMITY PAIN
crazy	CONFUSION*
cuts	ABRASION-LACERATION*
cyanosis	BREATHING TROUBLE* CYANOSIS*
dark urine	DARK URINE URINE TROUBLE
deaf	EAR PROBLEMS

* Potentially life threatening symptom

decrease sex	DEPRESSION SEXUAL PROBLEMS
decrease urine stream	URINE PROBLEMS
decrease vision	DOUBLE VISION EYE PROBLEMS
dehydration	DIARRHEA EXCESSIVE DRINKING-URINATION FEVER HEAT "STROKE"*
delirium	CONFUSION*
dementia	CONFUSION*
dentition	MOUTH TROUBLE
depression	ADOLESCENT-PUBERTY PROBLEMS DEPRESSION SUICIDE THOUGHTS*
dermatitis	ALLERGIES SKIN PROBLEM
diabetes	DIABETES
diaper rash	DIAPER RASH
diaper staining	DIAPER STAINING
diarrhea	ABDOMINAL PAIN* DIARRHEA
diet	EXCESSIVE EATING
difficulty swallowing	DIFFICULTY SWALLOWING
difficulty voiding	URINE TROUBLE
diplopia	DOUBLE VISION
disc	BACK PAIN
discharge ear	EAR PROBLEMS
discharge penis	VD

* Potentially life threatening symptom

SYMPTOM

discharge vagina	ABORTION* DISCHARGE VAGINA VAGINAL BLEEDING PROBLEMS VD
discoloration	CYANOSIS* PIGMENT CHANGE
dizzy-vertigo	BLACK OUTS* CONVULSIONS* DIZZY-VERTIGO GAIT-COORDINATION
double vision	DOUBLE VISION EYE PROBLEMS
dribbling urine	URINE TROUBLE
drinking	ALCOHOLISM EXCESSIVE DRINKING-URINATING
drooling	MOUTH TROUBLE
drowsiness	CONFUSION* UNCONSCIOUS-STUPOR*
drugs	see MEDICATION SHEETS OVERDOSE*
dysphagia	DIFFICULTY SWALLOWING
dysmenorrhea	CRAMPS-MENSTRUAL
dyspnea	BREATHING TROUBLE*
dysuria	DISCHARGE VAGINA URINE TROUBLE VD
ear problems	EAR PROBLEMS
eating - excessive	DIABETES EATING-EXCESSIVE OBESITY THYROID TROUBLE
eating too little	ANOREXIA
eczema	ALLERGIES SKIN PROBLEM
edema	SWELLING
elbow	HAND-WRIST-ARM PROBLEMS

* Potentially life threatening symptom

emotional trouble	ADOLESCENT-PUBERTY PROBLEMS BEHAVIOR-IRRITABILITY PROBLEMS CONFUSION* DEPRESSION HYPERACTIVITY SEXUAL PROBLEM SUICIDE THOUGHTS*
emphysema	ASTHMA BREATHING TROUBLE* COUGH
eneuresis	BED WETTING
epilepsy	CONVULSIONS*
epistaxis	NOSE-SINUS PROBLEMS
equilibrium	DIZZY-VERTIGO GAIT-COORDINATION
excessive drinking-urinating	ALCOHOLISM DIABETES EXCESSIVE DRINKING-URINATING URINE TROUBLE
exercise tolerance decrease	BREATHING TROUBLE* CHEST PAIN* DEPRESSION LETHARGY MUSCLE WEAKNESS
eye problems	DOUBLE VISION EYE PROBLEMS
facial pain	FACIAL PAIN HEADACHE NOSE-SINUS PROBLEM
failure to thrive	SICK FREQUENTLY SMALL BABY
fainting	BLACKOUT* CONVULSION* DIZZY-VERTIGO
fatigue	DEPRESSION LETHARGY MUSCLE WEAKNESS
fever	FEVER HEAT "STROKE"*
fits	CONVULSION*
flank pain	ABDOMINAL PAIN* BACK PAIN COUGH DARK URINE URINE TROUBLE
flatulence	INDIGESTION
flu	DIARRHEA NAUSEA AND VOMITING UPPER RESPIRATORY INFECTION

SYMPTOM

fluid	SWELLING
food poisoning	DIARRHEA
foot-ankle problems	FOOT-ANKLE PROBLEMS
fracture	FOOT-ANKLE PROBLEMS HAND-ARM-WRIST PROBLEMS HEAD INJURY* TRAUMA*
frequency	URINE TROUBLE
frigidity	SEXUAL PROBLEMS
frostbite	FROSTBITE*
fussy	BEHAVIOR-IRRITABILITY
gait coordination	BLACK OUT* DIZZY-VERTIGO GAIT-COORDINATION MUSCLE WEAKNESS NUMBNESS
gas	INDIGESTION
gastroenteritis	DIARRHEA NAUSEA-VOMITING
glands, swollen	LUMP-LYMPHADENOPATHY
glaucoma	EYE PROBLEMS
goiter	THYROID TROUBLE
gonorrhea	VD
gout	JOINT-EXTREMITY PAIN
growth	LUMP-LYMPHADENOPATHY
gum trouble	MOUTH TROUBLE
hair change	HAIR CHANGE

* Potentially life threatening symptom

hallucination	CONFUSION*
hand-wrist problems	ABRASION-LACERATION* HAND-WRIST-ARM PROBLEMS
hay fever	ALLERGY ASTHMA BREATHING TROUBLE* NOSE-SINUS PROBLEM UPPER RESPIRATORY INFECTION
headache	HEADACHE
head holding	FEVER HEADACHE
head injury	HEAD INJURY* UNCONSCIOUS-STUPOR*
hearing trouble	EAR PROBLEMS
heartburn	INDIGESTION
heart trouble	ANGINA* BREATHING TROUBLE* CHEST PAIN* PALPITATION
heat intolerance	THYROID TROUBLE
heat "stroke"	HEAT "STROKE"*
heaves	NAUSEA-VOMITING
hematemesis	VOMITING BLOOD*
hematuria	DARK URINE
hemorrhage	ABORTION* ABRASION-LACERATION* BLOOD IN STOOL* BRUISING-BLEEDING TENDENCY* VOMITING BLOOD*
hemoptysis	COUGHING BLOOD VOMITING BLOOD*
hemorrhoids	ANUS PROBLEMS
hepatitis	JAUNDICE*
hernia-abdominal	WELL BABY CHECK

* Potentially life threatening symptom

SYMPTOM

hernia-inguinal	HERNIA-INGUINAL
hesitancy	URINE TROUBLE
hiccough	HICCOUGH
hip pain	JOINT-EXTREMITY PAIN
hives	ALLERGIES SKIN PROBLEMS
hoarseness	DIFFICULTY SWALLOWING HOARSENESS TALKING TROUBLE
hot flashes	DEPRESSION VAGINAL BLEEDING PROBLEMS
hyperactivity	HYPERACTIVITY
hypertension	DEPRESSION (anxiety) HEADACHE HYPERTENSION
hypoglycemia	DIZZY-VERTIGO
imbalance	GAIT-COORDINATION
immunization	WELL BABY CHECK
impotence	SEXUAL PROBLEM
incontinence	BED WETTING URINE TROUBLE
indigestion	ABDOMINAL PAIN* INDIGESTION
infection	ABSCESS FEVER
infertility	INFERTILITY SEXUAL PROBLEM
injury	ABRASION-LACERATION* FOOT-ANKLE PROBLEM HAND-WRIST-ARM PROBLEM HEAD INJURY* TRAUMA*
insomnia	DEPRESSION LETHARGY

* Potentially life threatening symptom

irregular bowels	CONSTIPATION DIARRHEA
irregular periods	VAGINAL BLEEDING PROBLEMS
irritability	BEHAVIOR-IRRITABILITY HYPERACTIVITY
itching	ANUS PROBLEM SKIN PROBLEM

jaundice	JAUNDICE*
jaw	FACIAL PAIN
joint extremity pain	FOOT-ANKLE PROBLEMS HAND-WRIST-ARM PROBLEM JOINT-EXTREMITY PAIN

kidney trouble	DARK URINE URINE TROUBLE
knee	JOINT-EXTREMITY PAIN

laceration	ABRASION-LACERATION*
lactation	BREAST PROBLEMS
leg trouble	BACK PAIN FOOT-ANKLE PROBLEM JOINT-EXTREMITY PAIN ULCER, LEG
lethargy	DEPRESSION LETHARGY UNCONSCIOUS-STUPOR*
light headed	DIZZY-VERTIGO
light stools	JAUNDICE*
limp	GAIT-COORDINATION JOINT-EXTREMITY PAIN
lip trouble	MOUTH TROUBLE
liver disease	ALCOHOLISM JAUNDICE*

* Potentially life threatening symptom

SYMPTOM

loose stools	DIARRHEA
loss of appetite	ANOREXIA
lump-lymphadenopathy	ABSCESS BREAST PROBLEM LUMP-LYMPHADENOPATHY TESTICLE TROUBLE
lung trouble	BREATHING TROUBLE* COUGH COUGHING BLOOD
lymph node	LUMP-LYMPHADENOPATHY
malnutrition	ANOREXIA SWELLING WEIGHT LOSS
measles	FEVER SKIN TROUBLE
medication	see MEDICATION SHEETS
melena	BLOOD IN STOOLS*
memory problem	CONFUSION* DEPRESSION UNCONSCIOUS-STUPOR*
mental troubles	CONFUSION* DEPRESSION UNCONSCIOUS-STUPOR*
menorrhagia	VAGINAL BLEEDING PROBLEMS
menstrual problems	CRAMP, MENSTRUAL VAGINAL BLEEDING PROBLEM
migraine	HEADACHE
miscarriage	ABORTION*
missed period	PREGNANCY VAGINAL BLEEDING PROBLEM
mole	LUMP-LYMPHADENOPATHY
mononucleosis	LUMP-LYMPHADENOPATHY UPPER RESPIRATORY INFECTION
mouth troubles	MOUTH TROUBLES
multiple complaints	DEPRESSION (anxiety) specify the complaints

* Potentially life threatening symptom

mumps	LUMP-LYMPHADENOPATHY TESTICLE TROUBLE
muscle weakness	LETHARGY MUSCLE WEAKNESS STROKE*
myalgia	JOINT-EXTREMITY PAIN UPPER RESPIRATORY INFECTION
nail problems	NAIL PROBLEMS
nausea-vomiting	BLOOD IN STOOL* CHEST PAIN* NAUSEA-VOMITING VOMITING BLOOD*
neck trouble	NECK PAIN
nervous	DEPRESSION (anxiety) THYROID TROUBLE TREMOR
night sweats	FEVER
nipple problem	BREAST PROBLEM
no appetite	ANOREXIA
no energy	DEPRESSION LETHARGY
nocturia	BED WETTING BREATHING TROUBLE* URINE TROUBLE
nodule	LUMP-LYMPHADENOPATHY
noisy breathing	ASTHMA BREATHING TROUBLE*
nose trouble	NOSE-SINUS PROBLEMS UPPER RESPIRATORY INFECTION
numbness	BACK PAIN JOINT-EXTREMITY PAIN NECK PAIN NUMBNESS STROKE*
obesity	OBESITY

* Potentially life threatening symptom

SYMPTOM

oral problems	MOUTH TROUBLE
overactivity	HYPERACTIVITY
overdose	OVERDOSE*
orthopnea	BREATHING TROUBLE*
pain	specify: ABDOMINAL PAIN* ANGINA* BACK PAIN CHEST PAIN* CRAMPS, MENSTRUAL EAR PROBLEMS HEADACHE JOINT-EXTREMITY PAIN NECK PAIN TRAUMA* URINE TROUBLES
pale	ANEMIA
palpitations	ANGINA* PALPITATIONS
paralysis	MUSCLE WEAKNESS STROKE*
passed out	BLACKOUT* DIZZY-VERTIGO UNCONSCIOUS*
pelvic problems	ABDOMINAL PAIN* CRAMPS, MENSTRUAL DISCHARGE, VAGINA URINE TROUBLE VAGINAL BLEEDING PROBLEMS VD
penile discharge	VD
penile lesion	SKIN TROUBLE VD
period problems	CRAMPS, MENSTRUAL PREGNANCY VAGINAL BLEEDING PROBLEMS
petechiae	BRUISING-BLEEDING TENDENCY*
pigment change	PIGMENT CHANGE SKIN TROUBLE
piles	ANUS PROBLEMS
pimples	ADOLESCENT-PUBERTY PROBLEMS SKIN TROUBLE

* Potentially life threatening symptom

pleurisy	BREATHING TROUBLE* CHEST PAIN* COUGH COUGHING BLOOD
pneumonia	BREATHING TROUBLE* COUGH
poison	OVERDOSE*
poison ivy	SKIN TROUBLE
polydipsia	EXCESSIVE DRINKING-EXCESSIVE URINATION
polyuria	EXCESSIVE DRINKING-EXCESSIVE URINATION
post nasal drip	NOSE-SINUS PROBLEMS UPPER RESPIRATORY INFECTION
pregnant	PREGNANT
prominence of eyes	THYROID TROUBLE
prostate trouble	DARK URINE URINE TROUBLE
pruritus	SKIN TROUBLE
psychosis	CONFUSION*
puberty	ADOLESCENT-PUBERTY PROBLEMS
pulmonary problems	ASTHMA BREATHING TROUBLE* COUGH COUGHING BLOOD CYANOSIS* TUBERCULOSIS
pustule	ABSCESS SKIN TROUBLE
rash	SKIN TROUBLE
rectal bleeding	ANUS PROBLEMS BLOOD IN STOOL*
rectal problems	ANUS PROBLEMS BLOOD IN STOOLS* DIARRHEA
retardation	CONFUSION* RETARDATION

* Potentially life threatening symptom

SYMPTOM

red eye	DOUBLE VISION EYE PROBLEMS
red skin	SKIN TROUBLE
renal trouble	DARK URINE URINE TROUBLE
restlessness	CONFUSION DEPRESSION (ANXIETY) HYPERACTIVITY THYROID TROUBLE
rheumatic fever	BREATHING TROUBLE* FEVER JOINT-EXTREMITY PAIN
ringing in ears	DIZZY-VERTIGO EAR PROBLEMS
run down	DEPRESSION LETHARGY
runny nose	NOSE-SINUS PROBLEM UPPER RESPIRATORY INFECTION
salivation-drooling	MOUTH TROUBLE
scratch	ABRASION-LACERATION* SKIN PROBLEM
seeing difficulty	DOUBLE VISION EYE PROBLEMS
seizure	CONVULSIONS*
senility	CONFUSION*
sensation problem	JOINT-EXTREMITY PAIN NUMBNESS STROKE*
sexual problem	ADOLESCENT-PUBERTY PROBLEM BIRTH CONTROL INFERTILITY SEXUAL PROBLEM VD
shaking	ALCOHOLISM CONVULSION* TREMOR TWITCHING
short of breath	BREATHING TROUBLE*
shoulder trouble	ANGINA* CHEST PAIN* JOINT-EXTREMITY PAIN

* Potentially life threatening symptom

"sick"	specify nature of complaint DEPRESSION LETHARGY SICK FREQUENTLY
sick frequently	SICK FREQUENTLY
sick to stomach	NAUSEA-VOMITING
sinus problem	NOSE-SINUS PROBLEM UPPER RESPIRATORY INFECTION
skin problem	HAIR CHANGE LUMP-LYMPHADENOPATHY PIGMENT CHANGE SKIN PROBLEM ULCER, LEG
sleep trouble	DEPRESSION LETHARGY
small baby	SMALL BABY
sneezing	UPPER RESPIRATORY INFECTION ALLERGIES
sore-genital	VD
sore-other	SKIN PROBLEMS ULCER, LEG
sore-throat	UPPER RESPIRATORY INFECTION
speaking problems	DIFFICULTY SWALLOWING HOARSENESS STROKE* TALKING TROUBLES
"spells"	BLACK OUT* DEPRESSION (anxiety) DIZZY-VERTIGO
spine trouble	BACK PAIN NECK PAIN
spotting	ABORTION* VAGINAL BLEEDING PROBLEMS
sputum	COUGH
staggering	ALCOHOLISM GAIT-COORDINATION
sterility	INFERTILITY SEXUAL PROBLEMS
stiff neck	FEVER HEADACHE NECK PAIN

* Potentially life threatening symptom

DATA BASE PAGES AVAILABLE

SYMPTOM

stomach	ABDOMINAL PAIN* NAUSEA-VOMITING	INDIGESTION	
stones-gallstones	ABDOMINAL PAIN* STONES-GALLSTONES	JAUNDICE*	
stones-kidney	ABDOMINAL PAIN* URINE TROUBLE	DARK URINE	
stool	BLOOD IN STOOL* DIARRHEA	CONSTIPATION	
strabismus	DOUBLE VISION	EYE PROBLEMS	
strep throat	UPPER RESPIRATORY INFECTION		
stridor	BREATHING TROUBLE*		
"stroke"	STROKE*	UNCONSCIOUS*	
stuffy nose	NOSE-SINUS PROBLEMS UPPER RESPIRATORY INFECTION		
stupor	CONFUSION*	HEAD INJURY*	UNCONSCIOUS-STUPOR*
stuttering	TALKING TROUBLE		
sty	EYE PROBLEMS		
"sugar"	DIABETES		
suicide thoughts	OVERDOSE*	SUICIDE THOUGHTS*	
swallowing pain	DIFFICULTY SWALLOWING		
sweating	FEVER		
swelling	JOINT-EXTREMITY PROBLEM LUMP-LYMPHADENOPATHY	SWELLING	TRAUMA*
swollen glands	LUMP-LYMPHADENOPATHY		
syncope	BLACK OUT*		
syphilis	VD		

* Potentially life threatening symptom

talking trouble	HOARSENESS STROKE* TALKING TROUBLE
tantrum	BEHAVIOR-IRRITABILITY HYPERACTIVITY
temperature	FEVER
teeth	MOUTH TROUBLE
teething	BEHAVIOR-IRRITABILITY MOUTH TROUBLE
testicle trouble	TESTICLE TROUBLE
thirst	EXCESSIVE DRINKING-EXCESSIVE URINATION
throat trouble	BREATHING TROUBLE* MOUTH TROUBLE UPPER RESPIRATORY INFECTION
thrombophlebitis	JOINT-EXTREMITY PAIN
thyroid trouble	OBESITY THYROID TROUBLE
throwing up	NAUSEA-VOMITING
tic	TWITCHING
tingling	JOINT-EXTREMITY PAIN NUMBNESS
tinnitus	DIZZY-VERTIGO EAR PROBLEMS
tired	DEPRESSION LETHARGY
toothache	MOUTH TROUBLE
trauma	HEAD TRAUMA* TRAUMA*
tremor	ALCOHOLISM DEPRESSION (anxiety) THYROID TROUBLE TREMOR
tuberculosis	TUBERCULOSIS
tumor	LUMP-LYMPHADENOPATHY
twitching	CONVULSION* TREMOR TWITCHING

* Potentially life threatening symptom

SYMPTOM

ulcer	ULCER, PEPTIC
ulcer, leg	ULCER, LEG
ulcer, mouth	MOUTH TROUBLE
unconscious	CONVULSIONS* HEAD TRAUMA* OVERDOSE* UNCONSCIOUS-STUPOR*
upper respiratory infection	UPPER RESPIRATORY INFECTION
upset stomach	NAUSEA-VOMITING
urine trouble	BED WETTING DARK URINE DISCHARGE-VAGINA EXCESSIVE DRINKING-EXCESSIVE URINATING URINE TROUBLE VD
urticaria	ALLERGIES
vaccination	WELL BABY CHECK
vaginal bleeding	ABORTION* VAGINAL BLEEDING PROBLEMS
vaginal discharge	DISCHARGE-VAGINA VD
varicose veins	SKIN PROBLEMS SWELLING ULCER, LEG
VD (venereal disease)	VD
vertigo	DIZZY-VERTIGO
virus	DIARRHEA NAUSEA-VOMITING UPPER RESPIRATORY INFECTION
visual problems	DOUBLE VISION EYE PROBLEMS
voice trouble	HOARSENESS TALKING TROUBLE
vomiting	NAUSEA AND VOMITING
vomiting blood	VOMITING BLOOD*

* Potentially life threatening symptom

walking troubles	DIZZY-VERTIGO GAIT-COORDINATION MUSCLE WEAKNESS
wart	LUMP-LYMPHADENOPATHY
weak	DEPRESSION LETHARGY MUSCLE WEAKNESS
weight gain	DEPRESSION OBESITY SWELLING
weight loss	ANOREXIA DEPRESSION WEIGHT LOSS
well baby check	WELL BABY CHECK
wheezing	ALLERGIES ASTHMA BREATHING TROUBLE*
worms	ANUS PROBLEM
wound	ABRASION-LACERATION*
wrist problems	HAND-WRIST-ARM PROBLEMS

* Potentially life threatening symptom

MEDICATION PAGES

Listed below are some of the commonly used generic or brand name drugs. The color of the drug is listed when it might help in the differentiation of one product from others used in the treatment of the same condition. The color coding scheme is modified from the PHYSICIANS DESK REFERENCE.

Drug names were chosen to represent a cross section of drug types or medications having certain therapeutic indications. Generic drug names are expected to become more frequently used and are listed whenever possible.

Therapeutic Indication or Drug Types
Listed Alphabetically Below:

Allergies (anti-histamines)	Decongestants (see "allergies")	Headache	Skin care
Angina	Depression	"Heart" (cardiotonic)	Sleep (sedatives)
Antacids	Diabetes	Hypertension	Steroids (see skin care, arthritis, asthma)
Antibiotics	Diarrhea	Laxative	
Anticoagulents	Diuretic	Nausea-vomiting	Thyroid
Arrythmia	Epilepsy	Pain	Tranquilizers
Arthritis	Gastrointestinal (antispasmodic)	Parkinson's Disease	Vertigo (see nausea)
Asthma (bronchodilator)			
Birth Control			
"Breathing" see asthma, cough or "Heart"			
Cholesterol lowering			
Cough and expectorants			

MEDICATION PAGES

THERAPEUTIC INDICATION	GENERIC NAME	TRADE NAME	COLOR*	HOW SUPPLIED (ADULT)	FORM
Allergies	chlorpheniramine	Chlortrimeton	yellow	4 mg	tablet
			orange	12 mg	tablet
	diphenhydramine	Benadryl	pink/white	25 and 50 mg	capsule
	ephedrine	---	---	25 mg	tablet
	tripelennamine	Pyribenzamine	green	25 and 50 mg	tablet
Angina	isosorbide	Isordil	yellow	2.5 mg	tablet
			pink	5 mg	tablet
			white	10 mg	tablet
	nitroglycerin	---	orange	0.4 mg	tablet
	propranolol	Inderal	green	10 mg	tablet
			white	40 mg	tablet
	erythrityl tetranitrate	Cardilate	green	5, 10, 15 mg	tablet
	pentaerythritol tetranitrate	Peritrate	green	20 mg	tablet
Antacids	aluminum hydroxide	Amphogel	---	---	suspension
	calcium carbonate	---	---	---	powder
	aluminum hydroxide and magnesium hydroxide	Cremalin, Maalox, Mylanta	---	---	suspension
	magnesium hydroxide	Milk of Magnesia	---	---	suspension
	magaldrate	Riopan	---	---	suspension
Antibiotics	ampicillin	Penbriten	black/red	250 and 500 mg	capsule
		Polycillin	gray/red	250 and 500 mg	capsule

Generic name	Trade name*	Color	Strength	Form
cephalexin	Keflex	green/white	250 mg	capsule
		green/lime	500 mg	capsule
cloxacillin	Tegopen	red/black	250 mg	capsule
erythromycin	Ilosone	white/red	125 and 250 mg	capsule
		pink	500 mg	tablet
methenamine mandelate	Mandelamine	blue	1 gm	tablet
penicillin G	Pentids	green	500 mg	tablet
		white	200,000 and 400,000 units	tablets
phenoxymethyl penicillin	Pen Vee K	white	125, 250, 500 mg	tablets
sulfisoxazole	Gantrisin	white	500 mg	tablet
tetracycline	Achromycin V	yellow/blue	250 and 500 mg	capsule
	Tetrex	yellow/orange	250 mg	capsule
Tuberculosis				
ethambutol	Myambutol	white	400 mg	tablets
isoniazid (INH)	---	white	100 and 300 mg	tablets
rifampin	Rifadin	maroon/scarlet	300 mg	capsule
Other-				
griseofulvin	Fulvicin	white	125, 250, and 500 mg	tablets
metronidazole	Flagyl	white	250 mg or 500 mg	tablets
nystatin	Mycostatin	brown	500,000 unit	vaginal suppository
		yellow	100,000 unit	vaginal tablet
gamma benzene hexachloride	Kwell	---	---	cream or lotion

* Trade name colors. Generic name color may vary.

THERAPEUTIC INDICATION	GENERIC NAME	TRADE NAME	COLOR*	HOW SUPPLIED (ADULT)	FORM
Anticoagulants	warfarin	Coumadin	lavender	2 mg	tablet
			peach	5 mg	tablet
			yellow	7.5 mg	tablet
			white	10 mg	tablet
Arrhythmia	procaineamide	Pronestyl	yellow	250 mg	capsule
			orange/ white	375 mg	capsule
	propranolol	Inderal	orange/ yellow	500 mg	capsule
			orange	10 mg	tablet
			green	40 mg	tablet
	quinidine	---	---	200 and 300 mg	
	quinidine gluconate	Quinaglute	white	330 mg	tablet
Arthritis	aspirin	---	white	330 mg	tablet
	indomethacin	Indocin	blue/white	25 and 50 mg	capsule
	phenylbutazone	Butazolidin	red	100 mg	tablet
	prednisone	---	---	1, 2.5, 5, 10, and 20 mg	tablet
Gout	allopurinol	Zyloprim	white	100 mg	tablet
			orange	300 mg	tablet
	colchicine	---	---	0.5 and 0.6 mg	tablet
	probenecid	Benemid	yellow	500 mg	oblong tablet
	colchicine/ probenecid	ColBenemid	white	500 mg/0.5 mg	oblong tablet
Asthma (bronchodilators)	aminophylline	---	---	100 mg	tablet
				200 mg	tablet
				500 mg	suppository
	ephedrine	---	---	25 mg	tablets
					tablet

Generic name	Trade name	Color	Dosage	Form
cromolyn inhalant	Aarane, Intal	---	---	inhalant
ephedrine/ aminophylline	Amesec	orange/ black	---	capsule
theophylline with other substances	Quibron	yellow	---	capsule
	Tedral	white	---	tablet
isoproterenol inhalant	Isuprel	---	---	inhalant
prednisone	---	---	1, 2.5, 5, 10, and 20 mg	tablet

Birth Control Pills

These contain varying amounts of estrogens and progestens prescribed most often as C. Quens, Ortho Novum, Enovid, Ovulen, Oracon, Norlestrin, and Provest.

Cholesterol Lowering

clofibrate	Atromid- S	orange	500 mg	capsule
cholestyramine	Questran	---	---	powder
nicotinic acid	Nicobid	black/clear	125 mg	capsule
		green/clear	250 mg	capsule

Cough and Expectorants

glyceryl guaiacolate	Robitussin	---	---	liquid
potassium iodide	---	---	---	liquid

Cough suppressants

codeine	---	---	30 mg	tablet
dextromethorphan	Robitusin DM	---	---	liquid
terpin hydrate	---	---	---	liquid

* Trade name colors. Generic name color may vary.

THERAPEUTIC INDICATION	GENERIC NAME	TRADE NAME	COLOR*	HOW SUPPLIED (ADULT)	FORM
Depression (antidepressants)	amitriptyline	Elavil	blue	10 mg	tablet
			yellow	25 mg	tablet
			brown	50 mg	tablet
			red	10, 25, and 50 mg	tablet
Diabetes	insulin injections - (regular or semilente are quick acting while NPH and lente are of medium duration)				
	acetahexamide	Dymelor	white	250 mg	oblong tablet
			yellow	500 mg	oblong tablet
	chlorpropamide	Diabenese	blue	100 and 250 mg	tablet
	phenformin	DBI	white	25 mg	tablet
			blue/white	50 mg	capsule
	tolbutamide	Orinase	white	500 mg	tablet
	Tolazimide	Tolinase	white	100,250, and 500 mg	tablet
Diarrhea	diphenoxylate	Lomotil	white	2.5 mg	tablet
	kaolin/pectin	Kaopectate	---	---	suspension
	paregoric	---	---	---	liquid
Diuretic	chlorothiazide	Diuril	white	250 and 500 mg	tablet
	ethacrynic acid	Edecrin	white	25 mg	oblong tablet
	furosemide	Lasix	green	50 mg	oblong tablet
	hydrochloro-thiazide		white	20 and 40 mg	tablets
		Esidrix, Hydrodiuril	pink	25 and 50 mg	tablet
	spironolactone	Aldactone	---	25 mg	tablet

	Generic	Trade	Color	Dosage	Form
Epilepsy	diphenylhydantoin	Dilantin	yellow	50 mg	triangular tablets
			orange/white	100 mg	capsule
			pink/white	30 mg	capsule
	ethosuximide	Zarontin	orange	250 mg	capsule
	phenobarbital	---	---	15, 30, and 60 mg	tablet
	primidone	Mysoline	white	50 and 250 mg	tablet
	trimethadione	Tridione	white	150 mg	capsule
				300 mg	
Gastrointestinal (antispasmodic-anticholinergic)	atropine	---	---	0.3, 0.4, and 0.6 mg	tablet
	belladonna	---	---	---	liquid
	dicyclomine	Bentyl	blue	10 mg	capsule
				20 mg	tablet
	propantheline	Pro Banthine	pink	15 mg	tablet
See also: Tranquilizers (minor), Diarrhea, Laxative or Nausea-Vomiting					
Headache	caffeine/aspirin/barbiturate/phenacetin	Fiorinol	white	---	tablet
			green/lime	---	capsule
	caffeine/ergotamine	Cafergot	gray	---	tablet
	ergotamine	Gynergen	gray	1 mg	tablet
	methysergide	Sansert	yellow	2 mg	tablet
See also: Pain Relievers and Tranquilizers (minor)					

* Trade name colors. Generic name color may vary.

THERAPEUTIC INDICATION	GENERIC NAME	TRADE NAME	COLOR*	HOW SUPPLIED (ADULT)	FORM
Heart (cardiotonic)	digoxin	Lanoxin	yellow	0.125 mg	tablet
			white	0.25 mg	tablet
	digitoxin	Crystodigin	orange	0.5 mg	tablet
			pink	0.1 mg	tablet
			yellow	0.15 mg	tablet
See also: Angina, Arrhythmia, and Diuretic					
Hypertension	diuretic	see Diuretics			
	guanethidine	Ismelin	yellow	10 mg	tablet
			white	25 mg	tablet
	hydralazine	Apresoline	yellow	10 mg	tablet
			blue	25 mg	tablet
			purple	50 mg	tablet
	methyldopa	Aldomet	yellow	250 mg	tablet
	propranolol	Inderal	orange	10 mg	tablet
			green	40 mg	tablet
	reserpine	Serpasil	white	0.1, 0.25, and 1 mg	tablet
	guanethidine/ diuretic	Esimil	white	---	tablet
	methyldopa/diuretic	Aldoril	orange or white	---	tablet
	reserpine/diuretic	Regroton, Diupres	pink	---	tablet
	reserpine/ hydralazine/ diuretic	Serapes	pink	---	tablet

	Generic name	Trade name	Dosage	Color	Form
Laxative	bisacodyl	Dulcolax	5 mg	orange	tablet
	psyllium mucilloid	Metamucil	---	---	powder
	Dioctyl sodium sulfosuccinate (DSS)	Colace	50 mg	red	capsule
			100 mg	red/white	capsule
Nausea-Vomiting	dimenhydrinate	Dramamine	50 mg	yellow	tablet
	diphenhydramine	Benadryl	25 and 50 mg	pink/white	capsule
	prochlorperazine	Compazine	5, 10, and 25 mg	lime	tablet
	trimethabenzamide	Tigan	100 mg	blue/white	capsule
			250 mg	blue	capsule
Pain	acetaminophen	Tylenol, Nebs	325 mg	white	tablet
	aspirin	---	330 mg	---	tablet
	codeine	---	30 mg	---	tablet
	meperidine	Demerol	50 and 100 mg	white	tablet
	morphine	---	(intramuscular)	---	
	pentazocine	Talwin	50 mg	pink	tablet
	propoxyphene	Darvon	32 and 65 mg	pink	capsule
	Oxycodone/aspirin/phenacetin/caffeine	Percodan	---	yellow	tablet
	propoxyphene/aspirin/caffeine/phenacetin	Darvon compound - 65	---	red/gray	capsule
Parkinson's Disease	amantadine	Symmetrel	100 mg	red	tablet
	benztropine	Cogentin	0.5, 1, and 2 mg	white	tablet
	levodopa	Larodopa	100, 250, and 500 mg	pink	tablet
	trihexyphenidyl	Artane	250 mg	pink/white	capsule
			2 and 5 mg	white	tablet

* Trade name colors. Generic name color may vary.

THERAPEUTIC INDICATION	GENERIC NAME	TRADE NAME	COLOR*	HOW SUPPLIED (ADULT)	FORM
Skin Care	griseofulvin	Fulvicin	white	125, 250, and 500 mg	tablet
	tetracycline	Achromycin V	yellow/blue	250 and 500 mg	capsule
		Tetrex	yellow/orange	250 mg	capsule
	fluocinolone	Synalar	---	---	cream or lotion
	flurandrenolide	Cordran	---	---	cream or lotion
	hydrocortisone	---	---	---	cream or lotion
	triamcinolone	Kenalog	---	---	cream
	nystatin	Mycostatin	---	---	powder or cream
	tolnaftate	Tinactin	---	---	powder or cream or solution

See also:
Allergies

Sleep (sedative)	chloral hydrate	Noctec	red	250 and 500 mg	capsule
	diphenhydramine	Benadryl	pink/white	25 and 50 mg	capsule
	flurazepam	Dalmane	orange/creme	15 and 30 mg	capsule
	pentobarbital	Nembutal	yellow	30 and 100 mg	capsule
			orange/white	50 mg	capsule
	phenobarbital	Luminal	white	15, 30, 60, 100 mg	tablet
	secobarbital	Seconal	red	30, 50, and 100 mg	capsule

See also:
Tranquilizers (minor)

Thyroid

Thyroid replacement hormones vary widely in color and dose. When possible, the specific manufacturer must be identified and the pill matched with those shown in PHYSICIANS DESK REFERENCE.

	Generic	Trade name	Color	Dose	Form
'anti'-thyroid	propylthiouracil (PTU)	---	---	50 mg	tablet
	methimazole	Tapazole	white	5 and 10 mg	tablet
Tranquilizers (major)	chlorpromazine	Thorazine	brown or orange	10, 25, 50, 100, and 200 mg	tablet or capsules
	haloperidol-	Haldol	white	0.5 mg	tablet
			yellow	1 mg	tablet
			purple	2 mg	tablet
			green	5 mg	tablet
	perphenazine	Trilafon	white	2, 4, 8, and 16 mg	tablet
	thioridazine	Mellaril	green	10 and 100 mg	tablet
			purple	15 and 200 mg	tablet
			brown	25 mg	tablet
			white	50 mg	tablet
	trifluoperazine	Stelazine	blue	1, 2, 5, and 10 mg	tablet

* Trade name colors. Generic name color may vary.

THERAPEUTIC INDICATION	GENERIC NAME	TRADE NAME	COLOR*	HOW SUPPLIED (ADULT)	FORM
Tranquilizers (minor)	chlordiazepoxide	Librium	green/yellow	5 mg	capsule
			green/black	10 mg	capsule
			green/white	25 mg	capsule
	diazepam	Valium	white	2 mg	tablet
			yellow	5 mg	tablet
			blue	10 mg	tablet
	hydroxyzine	Vistaril	green/lime	25 mg	capsule
			green/white	50 mg	capsule
	meprobamate	Miltown	green/gray	100 mg	capsule
		Equanil	white	200 and 400 mg	tablet

See also:
Sedatives

HISTORY

Descriptors:

General Descriptors: refer to inside cover.
Aggravating factors: food, medications, alcohol, movement,
   position, bowel movements, emotional stress.
   Females (only): relation to menses.
Relieving factors: food or milk, antacids, medications,
   alcohol, position, bowel movements, eructation or passing
   gas.
Past treatment or evaluation: ask specifically about past
   x-rays -- barium enema, upper gastro-intestinal series,
   gall bladder x-rays.

Associated Symptoms:

Change in appetite or bowel habits; weight loss; jaundice;
fever/chills; chest pain; back pain; trouble breathing; cough;
prior chest or abdominal trauma; burning on urination; hematuria; dark urine; vomiting/vomiting blood; diarrhea; constipation (last bowel movement more than 24 hours ago); bloody or
tarry bowel movements.

Female patient: relation of pain to menstrual periods, vaginal
discharge, possibility of pregnancy, last menstrual period,
dyspareunia, abnormal vaginal bleeding.

Medical History:

Diabetes; arteriosclerotic heart disease (myocardial infarction or angina pectoris); atrial fibrillation; any prior abdominal surgery (was appendix removed?); kidney stones; gall
bladder disease; hiatus hernia; peptic ulcer; colitis; liver
disease.

Medications:

Aspirin; adrenal steroids; indomethacin (Indocin); alcohol
(more than a quart per week.)

Family History:

Colitis; ulcers; enteritis.

PHYSICAL EXAMINATION

Measure: temperature; sitting and lying blood pressure and
  pulse; weight.
Chest: asymmetric excursion, dullness to percussion, rales,
  rubs. Check for costovertebral angle tenderness.
Abdomen: tenderness, rigidity, abnormal bowel sounds, masses,
  aorta size, liver size.
Rectal: tenderness, masses. Test stool for blood.
Genital: Female, pelvic: adnexal tenderness, pain on cervical
  movement, uterine size and consistency, discharge from cervix, masses.
        Male: check for inguinal hernia.
Skin: rashes, bruises, jaundice, spider angiomata.
Pulses: femoral pulses.
Special, Psoas test: raise extended leg or hyperextend leg
  at hip. Does this procedure cause pain.
        Rebound tenderness: palpate the abdomen and then
  suddenly remove the palpating hand. Note if this causes
  pain. Note the location of the pain.
        Obturator test: flex and externally rotate the leg
  at the hip.Does this procedure cause pain.

DIAGNOSTIC CONSIDERATIONS	HISTORY	PHYSICAL EXAM
ACUTE ABDOMINAL PAIN, LIFE THREATENING:		
Peritonitis	Pain severe and gen-eralized; prostration; fever/chills; move-ment worsens pain.	Fever; generalized abdominal tenderness with guarding, rigidi-ty and rebound tender-ness; decreased bowel sounds; patient lies still; hypotension, tachycardia,pallor and sweating may be present.
Perforation of viscus	Pain severe and generalized.	Signs of peritonitis.

DIAGNOSTIC CONSIDERATIONS	HISTORY	PHYSICAL EXAM

ACUTE ABDOMINAL PAIN, LIFE THREATENING: (Continued)

Bowel Infarction | Patient is usually older than 50 years of age (unless arterial embolus is the causative factor). Pain is often diffuse and may not reach maximal intensity for hours; bloody diarrhea occasionally. | Hypotension, tachycardia, pallor and sweating may be present; signs of peritonitis; abdominal distension.

Bowel obstruction | Nausea, vomiting, often a preceeding history of constipation, abdominal distension; pain may wax and wane; history of abdominal surgery. | Abdominal distension with generalized tympanitic percussion; high pitched rushing bowel sounds early, decreased later; patient tosses and turns.

Rupture of an abdominal aortic aneurysm | Acute abdominal or flank pain. | Pulsatile abdominal mass; hypotension, tachycardia and asymmetrical pulses may be present.

ACUTE ABDOMINAL PAIN

Appendicitis | Initially pain is epigastric/periumbilical. Often progresses to right lower quadrant. Onset gradual, progressing over hours. | Low grade fever (less than 101° F); right lower quadrant tenderness on abdominal or rectal exam; bowel sounds variable; peritonitis if perforation occurs. Obturator psoas tests are often positive. Rebound tenderness referred to right lower quadrant.

Hepatitis | Malaise, myalgia, nausea and right upper quadrant pain. | Hepatic tenderness and enlargement. Jaundice may be present.

DIAGNOSTIC CONSIDERATIONS	HISTORY	PHYSICAL EXAM

ACUTE ABDOMINAL PAIN
(Continued)

Diverticulitis	Pain in lower left quadrant; constipation; nausea, often vomiting; course lasts several days. 25% of patients may have minor rectal bleeding.	Fever; lower left quadrant tenderness and fullness or mass; occasional rectal mass and tenderness; decreased bowel sounds. Localized signs of peritonitis may be present.
Cholecystitis	Colicky pain in epigastrium or right upper quadrant, occasionally radiating to right scapula; colicky with nausea, vomiting, fever; sometimes chills, jaundice, dark urine, light-colored stools (obstruction of common duct); may be recurrent.	Fever; right upper quadrant tenderness with guarding, occasional rebound; decreased bowel sounds.
Pancreatitis	Upper abdominal pain, occasionally radiating to back; mild to severe; associated with nausea/vomiting; history of alcoholism or gallstones; often recurrent; pain may be eased by sitting up or leaning forward.	Periumbilical tenderness; occasionally associated with hypotension, tachycardia, pallor and sweating; bowel sounds decreased.
Salpingitis (females)	Pain initially in lower quadrant but may be generalized; usually severe; fever/chills occasionally; dyspareunia; occasional vaginal discharge.	Fever; tenderness with guarding/rebound in lower quadrants; pain on lateral motion of cervix; adnexal tenderness; purulent discharge from cervix.

DIAGNOSTIC CONSIDERATIONS	HISTORY	PHYSICAL EXAM

ACUTE ABDOMINAL PAIN (Continued)

Ruptured ectopic pregnancy (females)	Last menstrual period more than 6 weeks previous; pain in one lower quadrant; acute onset and severe.	Adnexal tenderness and mass; postural hypotension and tachycardia may be present.
Ureteral stone	May note a history of previous "kidney stone"; pain may begin in flank and radiate to groin; painful urination and blood in urine are frequently noted.	Often unremarkable; flank tenderness may be noted as well as decreased bowel sounds. Fever is noted if urinary tract infection occurs.

CHRONIC ABDOMINAL PAIN

Reflux esophagitis	Burning, epigastric or substernal pain radiating up to jaws; worse when lying flat or bending over, particularly soon after meals; relieved by antacids or sitting upright.	Patient often obese; normal abdominal exam.
Peptic ulcer	Burning or gnawing, localized episodic or recurrent epigastric pain appearing 1-4 hours after meals; may be made worse by alcohol, aspirin, steroids or other anti-inflammatory medications; relieved by antacids or food.	Deep epigastric tenderness.

ABDOMINAL PAIN (ADULT)
(Continued)

DIAGNOSTIC CONSIDERATIONS	HISTORY	PHYSICAL EXAM
CHRONIC ABDOMINAL PAIN (Continued)		
Ulcerative colitis	Rectal urgency; recurrent defecation of small amounts of semi-formed stool; pain worsens just before bowel movements; blood in stools.	Low-grade fever; tenderness over colon; rectal tenderness and commonly blood in stools; weight loss may be present.
Regional enteritis	Pain in right lower quadrant or periumbilical; usually in young persons; insidious onset; may be relieved by defecation; stools are often soft and unformed.	Low-grade fever; periumbilical or right quadrant tenderness or mass; weight loss may be present.
Irritable bowel	Recurrent abdominal discomfort and/or change in bowel habits aggravated by anxiety; diarrhea often alternates with constipation.	No fever; minimal abdominal tenderness or normal abdominal exam; rectal examination is normal and feces contain no blood.

Reference: Harrison's Principles of Internal Medicine. 7th Edition, Pages 31-34.

HISTORY

Descriptors:

General descriptors: refer to inside cover.
Onset: acute or chronic.

Associated Symptoms:
Headache; coughing; vomiting; change in bowel habits; melena; weight loss; constipation; blood or worms in bowel movements; flank pain; hematuria; dysuria; joint pains; attention seeking behavior.

Family History:
Abdominal pain. Sickle cell disease.

Environmental History:
Child eats dirt or paint. Exposure to mumps or streptococcal infection in previous 3 weeks.

PHYSICAL EXAMINATION

Measure: pulse; temperature; blood pressure; weight.
Chest: rales; costovertebral angle tenderness.
Abdomen: tenderness; rigidity; abnormal bowel sounds; masses, liver size, spleen size.
Rectal: tenderness, masses. Test stool for blood.
Skin: turgor; dependent purpura.
Special: Psoas test: raise extended leg or hyperextend leg at hip. Does this procedure cause pain.
Rebound tenderness: palpate the abdomen and then suddenly remove the palpating hand. Note if this causes pain. Note the location of the pain.
Obturator test: flex and externally rotate the leg at the hip. Does this procedure cause pain.

DIAGNOSTIC CONSIDERATIONS	HISTORY	PHYSICAL EXAM
Acute Pain		
Appendicitis	Uncommon before the age of 3. Usually the pain is epigastric or periumbilical. It progresses to the right lower quadrant. The	Low grade fever (often less than 101° F). Right lower quadrant tenderness on abdominal or rectal exam is often noted; psoas/obturator

DIAGNOSTIC CONSIDERATIONS	HISTORY	PHYSICAL EXAM
Acute Pain		
Appendicitis	onset is gradual and progressive over hours. Vomiting and obstipation occur frequently.	tests are positive.
Mesenteric adenitis	Often the history is similar to above.	Temperature elevation (often more than 101⁰); right lower quadrant guarding is found less often than in appendicitis.
Henoch Schoenlein Purpura	Acute onset of joint, abdominal pains often progressing to severe vomiting and abdominal distention. Spontaneous bruising of skin eventually occurs.	Decreased bowel sounds; purpura in dependent areas.
Intussusception	Common at ages 5 months to 2 years; acute sudden abdominal pain, vomiting; decreased bowel movement often noted.	Mild temperature elevation; palpable abdominal mass may be present; high pitched rushing bowel sounds alternating with absent bowel sounds; blood may be present on rectal exam.
Bowel Obstruction	No bowel movement; vomiting, dehydration.	Increased bowel sounds initially; abdominal distention, hyperresonance, and decreased bowel sounds usually follows.
Pain from abdominal stress	Excessive coughing or vomiting causing diffuse abdominal ache.	Afebrile; minimal abdominal guarding.

DIAGNOSTIC CONSIDERATIONS	HISTORY	PHYSICAL EXAM
Subacute or Recurrent Pain		
Unclear etiology	Recurrent abdominal pain with no apparent damage to the child; headaches and vomiting are often claimed; possible attention seeking behavior.	Normal.
Constipation	Nonspecific abdominal ache.	Stool often palpable on rectal or abdominal examination.
Peptic ulcer	Nonspecific abdominal ache.	Stool often positive for occult blood.
Worm Infestation (Ascaris, Hook Worm, Taenia, Strongyloides).	Worms or ova may be noted in the stool; pain is frequently diffuse and not severe; weight loss, anemia and diarrhea may occur.	Usually normal exam. Pallor may be present in hookworm infection.
Renal disease (hydro-nephrosis, infection)	Pain often located in the flanks; hematuria or dysuria are sometimes present.	Occasional flank tenderness or masses may be present.
Colic	A problem of newborns often relieved by passing gas. Paroxysm of crying and writhing.	Increased bowel sounds during the attack.
Other Uncommon Causes of Abdominal Pain in Children		
Lead poisoning	Paint or dirt eating. Paroxysms of diffuse abdominal pain.	Usually normal.

DIAGNOSTIC CONSIDERATIONS	HISTORY	PHYSICAL EXAM
Other Uncommon Causes of Abdominal Pain in Children		
Sickle crisis	Black. Family history of sickle cell disease may be present.	Rigid abdominal wall; ileus.
Cholecystitis	See ABDOMINAL PAIN - Adult.	
Regional enteritis	See ABDOMINAL PAIN - Adult.	
Ulcerative colitis	See ABDOMINAL PAIN - Adult.	
Pancreatitis	See ABDOMINAL PAIN - Adult.	
Hepatitis	See ABDOMINAL PAIN - Adult	
Secondary to:		
Pharyngitis	Sore throat.	Fever; cervical lymphadenopathy, pharyngeal erythema.
Pneumonia	Cough; fever.	Fever; rales.
Mumps	Recent exposure to mumps.	Parotid gland swelling.

HISTORY

Descriptors:
  General descriptors: refer to inside cover.
  How long has the patient been pregnant; date of the last
  menstrual period; is there actual bleeding or merely spotting; how much bleeding (how many pads are soaked per hour
  or day); passage of tissue; duration of bleeding.

  Aggravating factor: was patient trying to induce an abortion;
  if so, how.

  Associated Symptoms: fever or shaking chill; lower abdominal
  pain or cramps; giddiness on standing.

  Medical History: previous abortion(s); history of previous
  pregnancies.

  Medications: any.

  Environmental: is patient married.

PHYSICAL EXAMINATION:
  Measure: sitting/lying blood pressure and pulse; temperature;
  respiratory rate.
  Abdomen: tenderness; uterine enlargement.
  Pelvic exam: masses; tenderness; any tissue passed; size of
  uterus and cervical os. (Pelvic examination in the third
  trimester is generally only recommended when an obstetrician
  is present.)

GENERAL CONSIDERATIONS:

Up to 20% of pregnancies abort before 20 weeks; there are
usually no apparent reasons for abortion.

The greater the amount of bleeding, the more likely the female
is to develop shock (orthostatic drop in blood pressure; pallor
and sweating); shock is a major risk during abortion.

ABORTION
(Continued)

DIAGNOSTIC CONSIDERATIONS	HISTORY	PHYSICAL EXAM
Septic abortion	Pregnant less than 20 weeks; often a history of trying to induce abortion; fever, chills and severe pelvic pain. The female is often unmarried.	Fever with abortion; exquisitely tender uterus or adnexae often present. Hypotension, pallor and sweating are frequently present.
Threatened abortion	Pregnant less than 20 weeks; vaginal bleeding; may have cramps.	Cervix is closed.
Imminent abortion	As above, but usually has cramps.	Cervix is dilated.
Inevitable abortion	As above.	Cervix is dilated; fetal or placental tissue is protruding from cervix.
Incomplete abortion	As above, but may have noted passing of tissue; cramps and bleeding persist.	Cervix is dilated; fetal or placental tissue may be present.
Complete abortion	Pregnant less than 20 weeks; fetal or placental tissue has been passed; cramps and bleeding have ceased.	omewhat variable, depending on time since abortion. Prompt closing of cervix expected after completed abortion.

DIAGNOSTIC CONSIDERATIONS	HISTORY	PHYSICAL EXAM
Placenta previa or abruptio placenta	Excessive vaginal bleeding during the third trimester.	Hypotension from blood loss may be present; fundus of uterus consistent with third term of pregnancy.

OTHER:

Bloody show	Minimal bleeding and passage of mucus plug prior to delivery; uterine contractions.	Term pregnant uterus.
Menstrual cramps	Non-pregnant woman; cramps and bleeding in association with menstrual period.	Normal pelvic exam.

For 'spotting'
or irregular
menses see (VAGINAL BLEEDING PROBLEMS)

HISTORY

Descriptors:

General descriptors: refer to inside cover.
Onset: when did injury occur; did it occur at work; type of
   trauma.
Aggravating factors: when was last tetanus booster; how many
   tetanus shots have been given in lifetime.

Associated Symptoms:

If injury to head: was there loss of consciousness. (if yes,
refer to TRAUMA).
If injury to chest: is there trouble breathing. (if yes, refer
to TRAUMA).
If injury to abdomen: any change in urine or bowel function.
(if yes, refer to TRAUMA).
If injury to extremity: any numbness or inability to move area
distal to injury. (if yes, refer to TRAUMA).

Medical History:

Diabetes; bleeding disorders; cardiovascular disease; connective tissue disease.

Medications:

Anticoagulants; adrenal steroids.

Environmental History:

Was the abrasion/laceration contaminated with feces, soil;
if animal bite, was attack unprovoked, what type of animal.

PHYSICAL EXAMINATION

Measure: blood pressure; pulse.
Skin: wound: size; location; crushed tissue, dirt, or foreign
   body in wound; if on extremity, check movement, sensation
   and pulses distal to injury.

GENERAL CONSIDERATIONS

Any wound is potentially contaminated with bacteria. Of
major concern is contamination with Clostridium tetani, a gram
positive bacillus which produces a toxin which affects the
spinal cord to produce severe, sustained muscle contractions
(tetanus). Clostridium tetani will not grow in the presence
of oxygen and requires a closed wound or necrotic tissue to
sustain growth and permit the secretion of toxin.

GENERAL CONSIDERATIONS

Prevention of tetanus can occur at three levels:

1. Growth of Clostridia in a wound can be prevented by thorough cleansing of the wound and removal of any necrotic tissue. The use of antibiotics in contaminated or neglected wounds is recommended to prevent growth of Clostridium tetani.

2. Patients can be stimulated by injection of tetanus toxoid to produce antibodies which will neutralize the tetanus toxin and prevent its action on spinal cord cells.

3. If there is a contaminated wound in a person who has never had tetanus immunization this person may be given tetanus antibodies from an immune person (tetanus immune globulin).

Extremity injuries may lacerate or sever peripheral nerves, tendons and vessels. If the patient has inadequate peripheral circulation they will heal poorly. Similarly, diabetes and connective tissue disease (particularly lupus erythematosis) affect small blood vessels and impair healing.

Wounds (especially stab wounds) to the chest and abdomen are particularly worrisome since underlying organs may be injured, and the extent of injury may be unclear at the time of initial evaluation. (see also TRAUMA).

HISTORY

Descriptors:

General descriptors: refer to inside cover.
Past treatment or evaluation: ask about previous treatment
and the results of this treatment.

Associated Symptoms:
Fever or chills; weight loss.

Medical History:
Recent surgery; previous abscesses; valvular heart disease;
connective tissue disease; diabetes.

Medications:
Adrenal steroids; antibiotics prescribed for abscess.

PHYSICAL EXAMINATION

Measure: temperature.
Skin: location of the abscess, size, and depth. Check for
fluctuance. Note if the abscess is on or near the following
areas: joints, hands, spine, nose, under arms, the perineum.
Nodes: check those draining the involved area.

GENERAL CONSIDERATIONS

Abscesses may be followed by severe systemic infections in
diabetics, in patients with connective tissue diseases (rheumatoid arthritis, systemic lupus erythematosis) and in those on
adrenal steroid medications. Abscesses in certain anatomical
areas (as noted above) can produce serious local complications.
Marked swelling and tenderness of lymph nodes often accompanies
early spread of the infection. Patients with valvular heart
disease are particularly susceptible to infection of the heart
valve. Fever, chills, and multiple abscesses may indicate
septicemia and probable valvular infection.

Reference: Harrison's Principles of Internal Medicine. Seventh
Edition. Pages 754 - 761.

HISTORY

Descriptors:

General descriptors: refer to inside cover.
Onset: when did the patient or parent first notice problem; what specifically is the problem.

Associated Symptoms:
Female: menses; vaginal discharge; breast development; slow development of secondary sexual characteristics.

Male: slow development of secondary sexual characteristics.

General: school problems; sexual dysfunction; drug abuse (cigarettes, alcohol, other drugs); masturbation; family problems; obesity; acne.

Medical History:
Any chronic diseases; past history of pregnancy.

Environmental History:
Nature of family, school and friends.

PHYSICAL EXAMINATION

Measure: blood pressure, height and weight.

Physical examination should be directed to those areas which are of concern to the adolescent (see other Data Base pages depending on the nature of the complaint).

GENERAL CONSIDERATIONS

The adolescent may suffer from the same problems as the child or adult, but because of the unique position of the adolescent any problem may have more psychological impact than otherwise. The adolescent often is unable to talk openly with experienced adults, so he/she must be reassured of the "normalcy" of mastur-bation, homosexual illusions, delayed puberty, menstrual irreg-ularities and pain or vaginitis. Concerns about birth control or venereal disease are not often discussed openly in school or at home. School failure is another often neglected problem for the adolescent.

The most common medical adolescent problems are obesity, vaginitis, acne, menstrual irregularity. Accidents and suicide

GENERAL CONSIDERATIONS

are frequent causes for adolescent death.

Puberty normally begins between 9 and 16 years of age. Endocrine dysfunction, brain tumors and genetic abnormalities often cause puberty to occur outside this expected range of normal.

HISTORY

Descriptors:

General descriptors: refer to inside cover.
Onset: age of onset of heavy alcoholic intake. Does patient
  drink to quiet nerves; drinking on job; morning drinking;
  number of drinks per day; last drink taken; longest period
  without a drink. In what form is alcohol usually taken.
Past treatment or evaluation: results of prior liver biopsy,
  upper GI series or liver function tests.

Associated Symptoms:

Shakiness; confusion; trouble walking; seizure; vomited
blood; dark black bowel movements; abdominal swelling; jaundice.

Medical History:

Seizures; delirium tremens; jaundice; liver disease; gastrointestinal bleeding.

Medications:

Anticonvulsants; aspirin; tranquilizers, antidepressants.

Family History:

Family history of alcoholism.

Environmental History:

Driving while intoxicated; arrests; loss of job; family attitude
toward drinking; family stability; do other family members
drink excessively.

False Positive Considerations:

If the patient is drunk, the history may be unreliable; in
general, alcoholics tend to minimize the amount and effects of
drinking.

PHYSICAL EXAMINATION

Measure: temperature; pulse; respiration; blood pressure.
Mental Status: carefully note the ability to recall recent
  events. Does the patient "make up" answers (confabulate).
Abdomen: liver size; ascites; spleen enlargement.
Extremities: tremor; asterixis (jerking motion on attempt to
  maintain a position).
Skin: spider angiomata; icterus.
Neurological: tandem walk; symmetry of reflexes; extra-ocular
  movements; vibratory sensation.

GENERAL CONSIDERATIONS

Drinking becomes alcoholism when the patient suffers a with-
drawal syndrome if alcohol is stopped, if the patient has
major alcohol associated illnesses, or if the patient demonstrates tolerance to alcohol (for example, the ability to
drink a fifth of a gallon of whisky or its equivalent per day
without becoming overtly intoxicated).

DIAGNOSTIC CONSIDERATIONS	HISTORY	PHYSICAL EXAM
Withdrawal syndromes:		
Tremulousness	Onset when patient awakes after several days of drinking; general irritability; gastrointestinal upset; patient needs to "quiet his nerves with a drink"; craves sleep.	Alert, easily startled; tachycardia, flushed skin conjunctival injection; rapid, coarse, often violent, tremor.
Delirium Tremens (DT's)	Fever; confusion; gross tremor; hallucinations within 1-3 days after cessation.	Fever; tachycardia; tremor; sweating; delirium; dilated pupils.
Seizures (Rum Fit)	Major seizure within 2 days of cessation of alcohol intake.	Major motor seizure; delirium tremens may also develop.
Major Alcohol Associated Diseases:		
Liver Disease	Jaundice; abdominal distention.	Spider angiomata; jaundice; ascites; liver and spleen enlargement may be noted. Increase in breast tissue is often present.
Bleeding Abnormalities	Vomiting blood; rectal bleeding or black bowel movements.	May have blood in stools and evidence for liver disease.

DIAGNOSTIC CONSIDERATIONS	HISTORY	PHYSICAL EXAM

Major Alcohol Associated Diseases:

Neurological Disease

	HISTORY	PHYSICAL EXAM
Subdural Hematoma	Fluctuating state of consciousness; often a history of previous head injury.	Hemiparesis or pupil abnormalities may be noted; neurological abnormalities may be <u>absent</u>.
Hepatic Encephalopathy	Abnormal mental status.	Severe liver disease; decreased mentation, asterixis, abnormal reflexes. Often progresses to coma.
Cerebellar Degeneration	Unsteadiness.	Nystagmus; ataxic gait.
Wernicke-Korsakoff Psychosis	Confusion; memory loss; heavy drinking without food intake for days to weeks.	Memory loss; nystagmus or loss of external gaze; confusion and disorientation; confabulation.
Neuropathy	Numbness or burning in feet and unsteadiness may be present.	Distal sensation deficit.

<u>Reference</u>: Harrison's Principles of Internal Medicine. Seventh
              Edition. Pages 673 - 681.

HISTORY

Descriptors:

General descriptors: refer to inside cover.
Aggravating factors: does contact with any substance, article or animal cause allergic symptoms.
Past treatment or evaluation: response to previous therapy (adrenal steroids, bronchodilators, antihistamines, skin creams, desensitization); results of past skin tests.

Associated Symptoms:
Rash; hives; insect bite; wheezing, trouble breathing.

Medical History:
Drug allergy (specify the type of reaction); asthma; eczema; hives; hay fever; food allergy.

Medications:
Adrenal steroids, bronchodilators; antihistamines; skin creams; allergy "shots"; antibiotics (tetracycline); decongestants.

Family History:
Asthma, eczema.

Environmental History:
Type of work; exposure to dusts, chemicals or animals; condition of housing and type of heating system. If insect bite: type of insect and past reactions.

PHYSICAL EXAMINATION

Measure: blood pressure; pulse; respiration.
Eyes: conjunctival injection or edema.
Nose: check nasal mucosa for polyps, secretions, mucosal swelling or pallor.
Chest: wheezing, distant breath sounds; prolonged expiration.
Skin: rash; (if insect bite, remove stinger).

GENERAL CONSIDERATIONS

At least 10% of the population suffers from "allergies." The most common complaints are rhinitis (sneezing, stuffy, runny nose, tearing and postnasal discharge) or asthma (wheezing and shortness of breath). Drugs, dusts, molds, foods, insect bites and skin contacts may precipitate rhinitis or

GENERAL CONSIDERATIONS

asthma; occasionally the skin responds acutely to the allergenic substance by the formation of hives, or less acutely by redness, scaling and oozing (eczema). Rarely acute reactions to allergens, particularly drugs and insect bites may cause a severe reaction manifested by hypotension, laryngospasm and wheezing (anaphylaxis).

One must determine:
1. Does the appearance of the allergic symptom follow any seasonal or known exposure pattern. Seasonal patterns often implicate pollens and molds as the cause: tree pollen--early spring; grass pollen--late spring; ragweeds--late summer; molds--all summer. (Temperate climates).

2. When and how is the allergy usually noted.

3. How has the allergy responded to past therapy. Have specific precipitating factors ever been proven and has avoidance of these factors caused improvement in the allergic symptoms.

Reference: Harrison's Principles of Internal Medicine. Seventh Edition. Pages 369 - 381.

HISTORY

Descriptors:

General descriptors: refer to inside cover.

Aggravating factors: cancer chemotherapeutic agents; 'gold' shots, chloramphenicol; mesantoin. Possiblity of arsenic, radiation or benzene exposure.

Past treatment or evaluation: why and when was the patient told that he is anemic; past examination of stool for blood; x-rays of bowels; bone marrow exam; blood tests.

Associated Symptoms:

Weight loss; weakness or dizziness when standing; petechiae; vomiting blood; black stools; greasy, foul smelling bowel movements or diarrhea; excessive menstrual bleeding (number of pads per day; number of days per month).

Medical History:

Bleeding disorder; sickle cell disease; hiatus hernia; peptic ulcer; gastric surgery; malignancy; alcoholism.

Medications:

Aspirin; adrenal steroids; iron; Vitamin B_{12}; folate.

Family History:

"Mediterranean" or Black ancestry.

Environmental History:

Precise description of how much milk, vegetables, meat and carbohydrates the patient eats; dirt or paint eating.

False Positive Considerations:

Patients who do not feel well for other reasons may claim that they are suffering from "low blood" while having no evidence for true anemia.

PHYSICAL EXAMINATION

Measure: weight; blood pressure and pulse lying and standing.

Eyes: conjunctivae - pink or pale.

Abdomen: liver, spleen size; masses.

Rectal: stool for occult blood; masses.

Extremities: vibratory sensation in toes; check palmar creases for pallor.

Skin: petechiae; ecchymoses; jaundice.

Special: a realistic evaluation of anemia should include, at the least, the measurement of the hematocrit and examination of a smear of the peripheral blood.

GENERAL CONSIDERATIONS

Anemia is found in many diseases. Most patients are found to be anemic by blood analysis, not by complaining that they are anemic. Anemia alone may cause the patient to feel weak and giddy, particularly if standing. As anemia becomes severe, the patient may be found to have orthostatic hypotension and tachycardia as well as pale palmar creases and conjunctivae. However, these symptoms and signs of anemia are often deceptively absent, and the chronically anemic patient may appear and feel normal.

The most common cause of anemia is iron deficiency. Iron deficiency anemia in the adult male or post menopausal female is presumptive evidence for a gastrointestinal source of blood loss and warrants appropriate evaluation before any treatment is given.

Anemia can be simply classified as a manifestation of inadequate intake of necessary hemoglobin precursors, of inadequate bone marrow production, or a manifestation of excessive blood destruction. Overlap between these general categories frequently occurs.

NOTE - evaluation of anemia is not realistic on the basis of the history and physical examination alone.

DIAGNOSTIC CONSIDERATIONS	HISTORY	PHYSICAL EXAM
Acute Blood Loss	Bleeding; tarry stools.	Orthostatic hypotension; pallor; stool often positive for occult blood.
Decreased Production by bone marrow		
1. Iron deficiency (Due to chronic blood loss).	The two most common sources of chronic iron loss are from the GI tract (tumor or ulcer) or from menstrual bleeding.	Stool may be positive for occult blood.

DIAGNOSTIC CONSIDERATIONS	HISTORY	PHYSICAL EXAM
Decreased Production by bone marrow		
2. Folate deficiency	Often alcoholism; poor nutrition, especially little meat or vegetables.	Often signs of alcohol abuse (see ALCOHOLISM).
3. B_{12} deficiency	Family history of anemia; chronic diarrheal disease.	Decreased vibration sense in toes.
4. Marrow Failure:		
Relative marrow failure	Chronic inflammatory disease, renal disease, infection, malignancy.	Signs of the chronic diseases are often present.
Marrow failure	Exposure to benzene, arsenic, or excessive radiation. Ingestion of chloramphenicol, mesantoin, gold shots or cancer chemotherapeutic agents.	Petechiae are often present.
Increased Destruction of red blood cells (sickle cell disease, malaria, G6PD deficiency, Rh or ABO incompatability).	Recent transfusion or a family history of anemia may be present. The parents of anemic newborn may have blood type incompatability.	Jaundice. Splenomegaly may be present.

<u>Reference:</u> Harrison's Principles of Internal Medicine. Seventh Edition. Pages 288 - 300 and 1580 - 1630.

HISTORY

Descriptors:

General descriptors: refer to inside cover.

Onset: number of episodes per day or week; has there been a change in the duration or frequency of the episodes.

Character: has there been a change in the character of the attacks.

Aggravating factors: anxiety; cold; deep breathing; meals; position; sexual intercourse; does pain come on at rest or during sleep.

Relieving factors: nitroglycerin ; antacids; cessation of exercise.

Past treatment or evaluation: how did the patient learn of the diagnosis of angina; previous exercise or resting electrocardiograms; past cardiac catheterization.

Associated Symptoms:

Palpitations; paresthesia in hands, fingers, or around mouth; nausea; trouble breathing; swelling of ankles; change in exercise tolerance.

Medical History:

High blood pressure; diabetes; obesity; intermittent claudication; elevated serum cholesterol or triglycerides; congestive heart failure; heart attack; cigarette smoking.

Medications:

Digitalis, diuretics; propranalol (Inderal); nitroglycerin ; long acting nitrates (Isosorbide).

Family History:

Atherosclerotic cardiovascular disease; high blood pressure; elevated cholesterol or triglycerides; diabetes; premature death.

PHYSICAL EXAMINATION

Measure: pulse, blood pressure.

Eyes: funduscopic evidence of arteriolar narrowing, arteriovenous nicking.

Chest: rales at bases.

Heart: gallops; enlarged or prolonged apical impulse; murmurs.

Extremities: edema; vascular insufficiency; lipid deposits over tendons.

Pulses: check all pulses for assymetry or absence; check for carotid bruit.

GENERAL CONSIDERATIONS

"Classic" angina implies the presence of exertional sub-
sternal chest pain radiating to the left arm, which is relieved by cessation of exercise or sublingual nitroglycerin
within several minutes. An S_4 gallop is frequently noted.
Only 50% of patients have all of these manifestations of
coronary artery disease, but, if all are present, the diagnosis
is virtually certain. Furthermore, an S_3 gallop present only
during pain is strong evidence that pain is due to myocardial
ischemia.

The approach to the patient involves the following considerations:
1. How much is the patient incapacitated.

2. Has there been a change in the quality, frequency or
duration of the pain, (unstable angina often precedes myocardial infarction).

3. What modes of treatment have been used and with what
result.

4. What other health problems may have contributed to the
development of coronary artery disease. Is there a family
history of atherosclerosis. Does the patient have lipid
abnormalities, hypertension, diabetes mellitus or aortic
stenosis. Is the patient a heavy smoker.

Reference: Harrison's Principles of Internal Medicine.   Seventh
             Edition. Pages 1194 - 1199.

HISTORY

Descriptors:

General descriptors: refer to inside cover.

Pediatric: does the child play with food; how much does the parent expect the child to eat.

Associated Symptoms:
Weight loss; nausea; vomiting; fever; abdominal pain; jaundice; joint pains; change in bowel habits; change in sleep or sex habits; decreased ability to concentrate; behavioral problems (pediatric).

Medical History:
Any diseases, particularly emotional, renal, cardiovascular, cancer, gastrointestinal; pediatric: cystic fibrosis.

Medications:
Note if any drugs are being taken.

Environmental History:
Unstable home environment; recent change in life style; pediatric: "forced" feeding.

PHYSICAL EXAMINATION

Measure: weight, height, temperature. (Pediatric: compare to growth chart standards).

A complete physical examination is usually recommended. Particularly emphasized are:

Chest: check for rales.
Heart: murmurs, rubs or gallops.
Abdomen: enlarged liver or spleen; masses; tenderness.
Extremities: wasting of muscles; edema.
Skin: jaundice; laxity and exaggerated wrinkling.

DIAGNOSTIC CONSIDERATIONS	HISTORY	PHYSICAL EXAM
Acute Disease (often gastro-enteritis or hepatitis)	Malaise; nausea; vomiting; abdominal pain; joint pains.	Usually normal; mild fever or jaundice may be present.

DIAGNOSTIC CONSIDERATIONS	HISTORY	PHYSICAL EXAM
Chronic Disease		
(Cancer, regional enteritis, alcoholism, kidney or heart disease. Also in children, cystic fibrosis).	Patient may note chronic abdominal discomfort, abnormal bowel habits, fatigue or breathing trouble.	Adults often show muscle wasting, laxity and exaggerated wrinkling of the skin; peripheral edema may be present. Children may show protuberant abdomen and wasted buttocks.
Psychological Cause		
(Depression; anorexia nervosa).	Patient may be depressed with disturbances of sleep, sexual function and inability to concentrate.	Weight loss may be present.
Drug Side Effect		
(particularly amphetamines)	Many drugs may cause anorexia.	Usually normal.
Parental Anxiety		
(Pediatric)	Normal children may show "fussiness" in eating; some parents worry about this.	Normal examination and growth parameters.

Reference: Harrison's Principles of Internal Medicine.   Seventh
             Edition.   Pages 210 - 211.

HISTORY

Descriptors:

General descriptors: refer to inside cover.
Aggravating factors: noted only during bowel movement.
Past treatment or evaluation: results of past rectal and/
  or sigmoidoscopic examinations; last stool examination
  for ova and parasites.

Associated Symptoms:
Pain; bleeding; burning; itching; swelling; prolapse; discharge; constipation; diarrhea; lack of bowel control;
worms seen in stool.

Medical History:
Hemorrhoids; liver disease; regional enteritis; ano-rectal
surgery; diabetes; past worm infestation.

Medications:
Rectal ointments; enemas; antibiotics.

PHYSICAL EXAMINATION

Rectal: examine for fissures, fistulae or hemorrhoids.
  Check stool for occult blood.
Special: anoscope examination.

DIAGNOSTIC CONSIDERATIONS	HISTORY	PHYSICAL EXAM
Hemorrhoids	Often very painful when thrombosis or when pro-lapse of hemorrhoids occurs. Bleeding may be noted on stools, toilet paper or in toilet water. Preg-nancy.	Hemmorrhoids. Internal hemorrhoid may be pro-lapsed through anal opening. A thrombosed external hemorrhoid is a tender, tense, smooth bluish elevation just beneath the skin.
Fissures or fistulae	Intermittent pain associated with bowel movement; itching, burning and purulent discharges; pain may lead to constipation;	Anal spasm; tenderness; rectal ulcers, fissure or fistulous openings are noted often near anal tags.

DIAGNOSTIC CONSIDERATIONS	HISTORY	PHYSICAL EXAM
Fissures or fistulae (continued)	fistulae are frequently observed in regional enteritis.	
Perirectal abscess	Extreme throbbing pain; perineal or perirectal swelling is frequently noted.	Localized perirectal redness and tender swelling.
Carcinoma/ polyp	Usually asymptomatic; change in bowel habits, blood streaked stools, or blood mixed with stool may be present.	Stool often positive for occult blood; a mass may be palpable on rectal exam.
Dermatitis (secondary to infection: yeast, pin-worms, amebiasis)	Itching is frequently noted; yeast infections are more common in diabetics and patients on anti-biotics.	The perianal area is red and often moist with blisters and crusts; white, curdy material may be present in yeast infection.
(Secondary to excessive scratching)	Often a "nervous habit" or due to poor hygiene. Persistent with no obvious infectious cause.	"Patches" of dermatitis.

Intestinal Parasites

Pin worms	Perianal itching.	Perianal skin inflammation.
Other - ascarasis, hookworm; strongyloidiasis, taenia	Often asymptomatic; worm may be coughed up, vomited or seen in bowel movement; abdominal discomfort and diarrhea occasionally present.	Usually normal.

HISTORY

Descriptors:

General descriptors: refer to inside cover.
Onset: what is the usual frequency and duration of attacks;
  are the attacks getting worse.
Aggravating factors: are attacks precipitated or aggravated
  by the time of year; known allergies or emotional stress.
Past treatment or evaluation: allergy tests; chest x-rays;
  respiratory function tests; results of past treatment. Has
  the patient been hospitalized for asthma.

Associated Symptoms:

Fever; purulent sputum; cough; chest pain; ankle swelling;
anxiety; confusion; lethargy; dyspnea.

Medical History:

Allergies to drugs; eczema; hay fever; cardiovascular disease;
emphysema; respiratory failure (requiring respirator, tracheal
intubation, tracheostomy).

Medications:

Adrenal steroids; bronchodilators; antihistamines; decongestants; allergy shots; antibiotics; inhalants; propranolol
(Inderal).

Family History:

Asthma; hay fever; eczema.

Environmental History:

Dusts; smoking; nature of occupation; possibility of inhaled
foreign body; atmospheric pollution.

PHYSICAL EXAMINATION

Measure: blood pressure (check for pulsus paradoxicus); pulse;
  respiration; temperature.
Nose: nasal polyps.
Neck: examine for tracheal deviation, venous distention and
  use of accessory muscles of respiration.
Chest: intensity of breath sounds; inspiratory to expiratory
  ratio; rales; ronchi; wheezes; check for unilateral hollow
  percussion note.
Heart: gallops; increased P_2.
Extremities: edema; cyanosis.

Pediatric: rib retraction; flaring of nostrils; cyanosis;
  stridor.

ASTHMA
(Continued)

GENERAL CONSIDERATIONS

Recurrent attacks of wheezing and shortness of breath are suggestive of asthma. However recurrent wheezing may be noted in emphysema, acute exacerbations of chronic bronchitis and congestive heart failure. The person with wheezing due to heart failure will usually improve with treatment of the failing heart.

1. An asthmatic with increasing symptoms must be evaluated to rule out infection, recent exposure to an allergen or pulmonary irritant, dehydration, or pneumothorax.

2. In the child under 6 years of age, wheezing (during colds) does not necessarily imply asthma. Infants with wheezing often have bronchiolitis and respond poorly to bronchodilator therapy.

3. Persistent wheezing in the adult or child may be due to a foreign body inhalation. (The wheezing is often localized).

4. Normal infants have noisy "rattling" breathing which is due to fluid in the upper airways.

5. There may be little wheezing in a severe asthma attack in which there is greatly reduced air flow in and out of the lungs. The person with severe respiratory failure may become anxious, confused or lethargic and have pulsus paradoxus on physical examination.

6. Propranolol is contraindicated in asthmatic patients.

Reference: Harrison's Principles of Internal Medicine. Seventh Edition. Pages 371 - 374.

HISTORY

Descriptors:
  General descriptors: refer to inside cover.
  Onset: did it follow direct trauma to back or fall from height.
  Location/radiation: be anatomically precise.
  Aggravating factor: coughing or sneezing; movement; menstruation.
  Relieving factor: antacids; leaning forward; bed rest.
  Past treatment and evaluation: spinal x-ray; spinal surgery;
    myelogram.

Associated Symptoms: urinary incontinence; inability to void;
  pain or numbness in buttocks or legs; abdominal pain; hip
  pain; dysuria, frequency or hematuria; fever or chills; nausea
  or vomiting; pain in costovertebral angle; vaginal discharge.

Medical History: history of malignancy; recent surgery or spinal
  fracture.

Medications: any regular medications, particularly adrenal steroids
  or anticoagulants.

PHYSICAL EXAMINATION

Abdomen: check for tenderness and masses. Check for flank punch
  tenderness. Check for bowel sounds.
Genital, female: if lower abdominal discomfort, relation of pain to
  menses or vaginal discharge. Do physical examination checking
  for tenderness or masses.
Extremities and back: check for spasm of paraspinous muscles, direct
  and sacroiliac tenderness, loss of normal lumbar lordosis and
  extent of spinal flexion when the patient bends forward.
Neurological, reflexes: ankle jerks, knee jerks and plantar reflex.
  Sensation: pinprick and/or vibration over large toe (L_5), small
  toe (S_1) and medial calf (L_4). Strength: have patient walk
  on heels and toes.
Special: perform straight leg raising test on both legs with knees
  fully extended. Note if straight leg raising causes or increases
  the patient's complaint of discomfort in the back, buttocks or
  legs.

GENERAL CONSIDERATIONS

It is useful to distinguish three kinds of back pain:

1) Pain of musculo-skeletal origin usually results from low back
   strain of muscle spasm, but may also be due to bony destruction, for example that due to tumor, osteomyelitis or vertebral
   fracture.

2) Diseases of the pelvic or abdominal viscera may produce pain
   which is referred to the back.

3) Radicular pain is due to the irritation of spinal sensory nerve
   roots, usually by herniated intervertebral discs.

Low back strain characterized by chronic recurrent low back
aching without neurological abnormality is the commonest form
of back pain. The major concerns in approaching the patient
with back pain are:

   1) Are major neurological deficits present or likely to occur?
   2) What potentially dangerous diseases might be causing the
      back pain?

DIAGNOSTIC CONSIDERATION	HISTORY	PHYSICAL EXAM
MUSCULOSKELETAL:		
Spinal fracture	Severe pain often following direct trauma to back or fall from height on to buttocks; older patients are at risk for fracture from minimal trauma; risk is enhanced in person taking adrenal steroids.	Localized spinal or paraspinal tenderness; neurological changes may be present.

DIAGNOSTIC CONSIDERATION	HISTORY	PHYSICAL EXAM
MUSCULOSKELETAL: (Continued)		
Osteomyelitis	May have a history of possible septic focus and fever (recent urinary tract infection or abdominal surgery); back pain constant and often progressive over weeks.	Spinal percussion usually produces pain; little or no fever.
Malignant tumor in vertebrae	Often severe progressive pain in older patient or patient with history of malignancy or weight loss.	Direct spinal tenderness to palpation and percussion.
Muscle strain	Often begins after lifting; no radiation of pain to legs.	Paraspinous muscle spasm; straight leg raising test does not produce back pain; no neurological deficit.
Osteoarthritis	Older patient; pains in other joints frequently present.	Limited range of motion of spine may be present.
Ankylosing spondylitis	Stiffness and low back pain usually in the young male.	Sacroiliac tenderness; reduced flexion of spine on forward flexion; loss of lumbar lordosis.

DIAGNOSTIC CONSIDERATION	HISTORY	PHYSICAL EXAM
VISCERAL:	Usually a history of abdominal pain and:	
Penetrating peptic ulcer	History of peptic ulcer; pain in back above lumbar area; pain often relieved by antacids.	Stool often positive for occult blood; epigastric tenderness.
Pancreatitis	Pain often relieved by leaning forward; upper epigastric discomfort; history of alcoholism or gallstones.	Epigastric or generalized abdominal tenderness; decreased bowel sounds.
Abdominal aortic aneurysm	Upper abdominal discomfort; patient usually over 50 years.	May have absent femoral pulses; palpable pulsatile abdominal mass usually present.
Renal disease (usually infection or renal stone)	Flank pain that may radiate to the perineum; dysuria or hematuria; fever may be present.	Flank or upper abdominal tenderness.
Gynecological disease	Lower abdominal or sacral discomfort; vaginal discharge; may note relationship to menstruation.	Abnormal pelvic exam.

DIAGNOSTIC CONSIDERATION	HISTORY	PHYSICAL EXAM
RADICULAR:		
Major neurological deficit	Often follows trauma with spinal fracture; may have insidious onset if secondary to tumor or herniated intervertebral disc; patient will sometimes note abnormalities of bladder function, inability to move legs or pain radiating to legs.	Bladder still enlarged after voiding; flaccid anal sphincter; sensory loss in perineum; absent deep tendon reflexes with demonstrable weakness and sensory loss in the extremities; plantar reflexes may be extensor if the spinal cord itself is injured.
Herniated intervertebral disc	Often pain began after lifting; pain usually radiates into leg(s) or buttocks(s); pain intensified by coughing, sneezing.	Decreased ankle or knee deep tendon reflexes; straight leg raising usually causes back pain at less than 60 degrees.
OTHER:		
Herpes Zoster (Shingles)	Older patient; underlying malignancy or other disease common; unilateral pain in girdling radiation.	Usually associated with skin lesions in a narrow (dermatome) band.

Reference: Harrison's Principles of Internal Medicine. Seventh
            Edition. Pages 34 - 43.

HISTORY

Descriptors:

General descriptors: refer to inside cover.
Present age of child; frequency of bed wetting; is child incontinent during the day or just at night; has the child ever been completely free of enuresis.

Associated Symptoms:
Polydipsia; polyphagia; polyuria; dysuria; seizures; numbness or weakness; emotional problems; dribbling urine or weak urine stream; sleep disturbances; discipline problems.

Medical History:
Diabetes; seizures; kidney diseases.

Family History:
Enuresis; diabetes.

Environmental:
Recent birth of siblings; other change in home environment.

PHYSICAL EXAMINATION

Abdomen: masses.
Neurological: perineal sensation and general neurological examination.
Special: developmental skills appropriate to the child's age.

GENERAL CONSIDERATION

Persistent inability to control urination during the day is not common and complete evaluation is usually indicated. On the other hand, sporadic enuresis may be seen in 10-20% of children up to age 10 and 1% of adult males.

DIAGNOSTIC CONSIDERATION	HISTORY	PHYSICAL EXAM
Psychogenic	"Emotional problems"; recent birth of sibling in older age children; family history of enuresis; daytime control.	Normal.
Diabetes or renal disease	Polydipsia; polyuria; dysuria; dribbling urine.	Often normal exam; occasionally enlarged kidneys or bladder.
Neurological disease	History of deficient developmental skills may be noted.	Neurological abnormalities frequently present. Developmental skills may be inadequate.
Seizures	Seizures or convulsive activity preceeding enuresis.	May be normal except during seizure.
Normal	Normal child with no history compatible with other causes listed above. Age usually less than 3-10 years.	Normal.

HISTORY

Descriptors:

General descriptors: refer to inside cover.
Age of child; what won't child eat or do normally; what is
the nature of the irritable behavior; is the child always
irritable or is present behavior an acute change; how does
the behavior differ from siblings at comparable age.

Associated Symptoms:

Headache or head holding; stiff neck; fever; ear pulling;
salivation; nausea; vomiting or excessive regurgitation; change
in appetite; loose stool; crying on urination; cough; wheeze;
trouble breathing; skin rash; change in weight; excessive
crying; reading difficulty; dislike of school; "clumsiness";
hyperactivity.

Medical History:

Any past diseases; birth trauma; retardation; seizure disorder.

Medications:

Any.

Environmental:

Change in life style of parents at home; change in diet;
change in school; attitude of others toward child; recent
birth of sibling.

PHYSICAL EXAMINATION

Measure: temperature, height, weight.
Head: fontanel for bulging.
Ears: check hearing; inner ear for inflammation.
Eyes: visual acuity (when possible).
Throat: check for inflammation.
Mouth: evidence of new teeth (infant).
Lungs: rales.

PHYSICAL EXAMINATION
(Continued)

> Heart: murmurs.
> Abdomen: masses.
> Neurological: general neurological examination.
> Special: check developmental skills appropriate to the
>   child's age.

GENERAL CONSIDERATIONS

Irritabilty, fussiness or a change in behavior may be noted in
any person -- particularly a child -- who does not feel well
and has underlying disease. Complete examination, particularly
to rule out meningeal irritation (stiff neck, bulging fontanel)
must be undertaken in the child with a recent change in behavior.

DIAGNOSTIC CONSIDERATION	COMMON CONCERNS
Behavior change secondary to underlying disease:	
Acute	Meningitis; viral disease; ear infection; hunger or teething (infant).
Chronic	Seizure disorder; dyslexia; asthma; minimal brain disfunction; poor hearing or vision; any chronic disease.
Behavior change secondary to reactions to chronic disease	Dysfiguring skin disease; deformity; mental retardation.
Primary behavioral disorders	Schizophrenia; autism; hyperkinesis syndrome (see HYPERACTIVITY).

HISTORY

Descriptors:

General descriptors: refer to inside cover.
Aggravating factor: what is the patient's motivation for
  birth control; what is the partner's attitude toward
  birth control; if adolescent, is parental consent required
  by local or state law.
Past treatment and evaluation: what methods have been used
  in the past; what were the results; past abortions or pregnancies.

Associated Symptoms:

Vaginal bleeding; vaginal discharge; headaches; menstrual
period overdue.

Medical History:

Regularity of menstrual periods; thrombophlebitis; pulmonary
embolus; cerebrovascular disease; cancer of breasts or reproductive organs; liver disease; migraine headaches; diabetes;
epilepsy; hypertension; uterine leiomyomas (fibroids); severe
depression.

Medications:

Any chronic medications.

PHYSICAL EXAMINATION

Measure: blood pressure.
Chest; breasts and axilla: check carefully for masses.
Genital; pelvic exam: check carefully for uterine masses,
  adnexal tenderness, cervical softening, color of cervix
  and uterine enlargement; do Pap test.

GENERAL CONSIDERATIONS

Oral contraceptives and intra-uterine devices are presently
two of the most popular methods of birth control. The intra-
uterine device should not be inserted when the patient is pregnant or has vaginal bleeding, vaginal discharge of undetermined

GENERAL CONSIDERATIONS
(Continued)

cause or uterine leiomyomas. Oral contraceptives have many side effects, interact with many medications and possibly accelerate the growth of breast or reproductive organ tumors.

RELATIVE EFFECTIVENESS	METHOD OF BIRTH CONTROL	COMMENTS
Poor	Postcoital douche, rhythm method, coitus interruptus.	Generally ineffective.
Fair	Spermicides with diaphragm, or condom.	Must be used every time; generally inconvenient but safe.
Effective	Intrauterine device	May be expelled spontaneously; pain, bleeding and infection may occur; 20% of patients must discontinue use because of side effects.
	Vasectomy or tubal ligation	Permanent sterility.
	Birth Control Pills	Contraindications for use include: thrombophlebitis, pulmonary embolus, cerebrovascular disease, cancer of breasts or reproductive organs, liver disease, undiagnosed vaginal bleeding; may also aggravate hypertension, epilepsy, diabetes, migraine headaches or growth of uterine leiomyomas.

HISTORY

Descriptors:

General descriptors: refer to inside cover.
Onset: was anyone present who observed the patient's black out spell; what happened; what position was the person in when he "blacked out".
Aggravating factors: cough; urination; turning the head; exertion; painful stimuli; fright; did patient strike his head.

Associated Symptoms: (occuring before or after syncope)
Seizure; visual changes; changes in sensation or ability to move; loss of control of bowel or urinary function; chest pain; hunger; sweating; black bowel movements; dizziness when standing.

Medical History:
Seizures; any neurological disease; diabetes; cardiovascular disease; chronic obstructive pulmonary disease.

Medications:
Digitalis; antiarrhythmics; anticonvulsants; antidepressants; antihypertensives; insulin; oral hypoglycemic agents.

False Positive Considerations:
The patient may claim that he "blacked out" whereas he really felt faint or giddy and never lost consciousness.

PHYSICAL EXAMINATION

Measure: blood pressure; pulse: lying and standing.
Heart: murmurs, gallops, arrhythmia; check apical pulse if pulse is irregular.
Rectal: stool for occult blood.
Pulses: check strength of carotid pulses; listen for carotid and vertebral bruit.
Neurological: sensation and strength of all extremities; deep tendon reflexes and plantar response; cranial nerve function.

GENERAL CONSIDERATIONS

Patients complaining of "black out spells" have often not
lost consciousness, but rather have experienced giddiness
(see Dizzy-Vertigo). Patients who actually do lose consciousness have often suffered from common fainting (vasovagal syncope)
following emotional stress or painful stimulation to the patient.

DIAGNOSTIC CONSIDERATIONS	HISTORY	PHYSICAL EXAM
Vasovagal/postural syncope (inadequate venous return to heart)	Syncope following emotional stress or bodily injury; syncope following standing, coughing or urinating.	Usually no abnormalities. Occasional orthostatic hypotension is present.
Syncope secondary to insufficient cardiac output (Stokes Adams Attacks).	History of heart disease, chest pain, or arrhythmias frequently noted; may follow exercise.	Cardiac exam reveals arrhythmias, slow heart rate or significant aortic stenosis.
Syncope secondary to cerebrovascular disease	Patients may notice sudden "drop attacks" with occasional residual changes in vision, speech, movement or sensory functions. This type of syncope may rarely occur following head turning.	May have neurological deficit; vertebral and carotid bruit rarely noted.
Syncope following blood loss	Black bowel movements may be noted.	Stool is often positive for occult blood; orthostatic hypotension and tachycardia are present.

DIAGNOSTIC CONSIDERATIONS	HISTORY	PHYSICAL EXAM
Medication related syncope:		
Guanethidine	Fainting on standing.	Orthostatic hypotension.
Digitalis	Aggravated by diuretics without potassium replacement.	Extrasystoles may be apparent on cardiac examination. Pulse rate may be less than 60 beats per minute.
Insulin or oral hypoglycemic agent.	Hunger, sweating, heart pounding before syncope.	The patient may become comatose.
Loss of consciousness during a seizure simulating syncope	Convulsive movements; loss of bowel or bladder control frequently occur.	Residual neurological abnormalities may be noted; soiled undergarments.
Psychological	Often unclear onset and prolonged "coma" without apparent cause; may fall but is seldom injured.	Eyelid fluttering may be noted despite the patient's overall appearance of unconsciousness.

Reference: Harrison's Principles of Internal Medicine. Seventh
            Edition. Pages 72 - 78.

HISTORY

Descriptors:
General Descriptors: refer to inside cover.
Character: is blood mixed through bowel movements; is
   toilet bowl water red or does blood only streak the
   stool or toilet paper; are any movements black or
   tarry.
Past treatment or evaluation: barium enema, upper GI
   x-ray or proctoscope exam done in past; results.

Associated Symptoms:
Abdominal pain; change in bowel habits; change in caliber
   of stools; mucus or pus with stool; painful bowel movements; nausea or vomiting; heartburn; vomiting blood;
   easy bruising; weight loss.

Medical History:
Hemorrhoids; diverticulosis; colitis; peptic ulcers;
   bleeding tendency; alcoholism.

Medications:
Warfarin (Coumadin); adrenal steroids; aspirin; indomethacin (Indocin).

Family History:
Bleeding problems.

False Positives:
The following substances may change stool color: beets,
   red; iron pills, black; bismuth (peptobismol), black.

PHYSICAL EXAM

Measure: blood pressure and pulse, sitting and lying.
Abdomen: tenderness, masses, ascites, hepatosplenomegaly.
Rectal: hemorrhoids, stool for occult blood.
Skin: spider angiomata, bruises, jaundice.

DIAGNOSTIC CONSIDERATIONS	HISTORY	PHYSICAL EXAM
UPPER GASTROINTESTINAL BLEEDING		
	Black tarry bowel movements (nothing but blood gives the stool a tarry consistency) often with vomiting <u>AND</u>:	
Peptic ulcer	Epigastric pain; history of aspirin or steroid ingestion; pain often relieved by food or antacids.	Epigastric tenderness.
Gastritis	Epigastric pain; excessive alcohol intake often preceeds onset of pain or bleeding.	Possible epigastric tenderness.
Esophageal varices	History of chronic alcoholism and/or liver disease usually present; vomiting blood common.	Spider angiomata; icterus; ascites; gynecomastia; splenomegaly.
LOWER GASTROINTESTINAL CAUSES FOR BLOOD IN STOOLS		
Hemorrhoids/ anal fissures	Minimal bleeding, often only blood streaking on stool of toilet paper; rectal pain may be noted.	Hemorrhoids and abnormal rectal exam.
Diverticular disease	Usually bright red blood with minimal **discomfort.**	Usually normal.

DIAGNOSTIC CONSIDERATIONS	HISTORY	PHYSICAL EXAM

LOWER GASTROINTESTINAL CAUSES FOR BLOOD IN STOOLS
(Continued)

DIAGNOSTIC CONSIDERATIONS	HISTORY	PHYSICAL EXAM
Ulcerative colitis; salmonella gastroenteritis; (tropical schistosomiasis and worm infestation); granulomatous colitis.	Abdominal discomfort; loose stools or diarrhea; pus in bowel movements.	Occasional diffuse lower abdominal tenderness and fever.
Intestinal tumors or polyps	May have weight loss, pain; usually not large amount of bleeding; change in bowel habits and caliber of stools.	Weight loss; palpable mass occasionally.
Gastrointestinal bleeding secondary to generalized bleeding tendency.	Melena or red blood; prolonged and excessive bleeding from scratches or lacerations; patient may be ingesting anticoagulents.	Skin may reveal large bruises or petechiae.

References: Harrison's Principles of Internal Medicine. Seventh Edition. Pages 244-246.

PEDIATRIC CONSIDERATIONS	FINDINGS	USUAL FREQUENCY
NEWBORN PERIOD		
Hemorrhagic disease of newborn	Evidence of bruising or bleeding disorder; bright red blood or melena.	Relatively common if vitamin K not given at birth.
Swallowed blood	Normal exam; often from mother's nipple or at deliveries; usually melena.	Common.
OTHER AGES		
Anal fissures, rectal polyps	Cause may be visible or palpable on rectal exam; blood usually streaks stool and is red.	Common.
Constipation	During bouts of constipation; bright red blood on stool.	Common.
Volvulus; intussusception	Abdominal pain; vomiting; decrease bowel movement.	Rare.
Meckels Diverticulum	No pain.	Rare.

Other considerations listed above as <u>adult considerations</u> are relatively uncommon causes of blood in the stool of a child.

HISTORY

Descriptors:

General descriptors: refer to inside cover.
Onset: date of first complaint.
Aggravating factors: relation of complaint to menses; last
  menstrual period; nursing; recent trauma.

Associated Symptoms:

Breast enlargement, pain, discharge (bloody or otherwise), or
mass; change in skin color or skin retraction on the breast;
excessive milk production; axillary swelling or lumps; fever
or chills.

Medical History:

Pregnancy; tuberculosis; known neurological disease; breast
cancer; benign cystic disease; alcohol abuse; liver disease.

Medications:

Oral contraceptives; phenothiazines; spironolactone (Aldactone);
diphenylhydantoin (Dilantin).

Family History:

Breast problems.

PHYSICAL EXAMINATION

Chest: breasts and axillary lymph nodes.
Genital: males: check testes for size and firmness.

DIAGNOSTIC CONSIDERATIONS	HISTORY	PHYSICAL EXAM
Breast enlargement (adolescent)	The male or female near puberty may have unilateral or bilateral enlargement.	Normal except for increase in breast tissue.
Breast enlargement (adult male)		
Liver Disease	Usually a history of chronic alcoholism.	Small soft testicles; jaundice; ascites; splenomegaly.

DIAGNOSTIC CONSIDERATIONS	HISTORY	PHYSICAL EXAM
Breast enlargement (adult male)		
Testicular Cancer	Asymptomatic testicular mass.	Firm testicular mass.
Drug Related	Chronic ingestion of spironolactone, diphenylhydantoin or estrogens.	Usually normal except for increase in breast tissue.
Breast Mass:		
Presumptive carcinoma	Family history of breast cancer may be noted; nipple discharge rarely present.	Axillary node enlargement; unilateral mass with ill defined border, fixation to surrounding tissue may cause dimpling of overlying skin.
Cystic mastitis	Multiple masses in the breasts usually becoming painful before each menstrual period.	Lumpy breasts with none of the characteristics of cancer listed above.
Breast pain:		
Hormonal engorgement	Pain and tenderness during early pregnancy or premenstrual cycle; oral contraceptives may aggravate the complaint.	May have "lumpy breasts" as above; usually normal.
Mastitis	Acute fever; tender swollen breasts; discharge. May follow trauma. Mastitis is more common in nursing females.	Localized breast tenderness, redness and fever.

DIAGNOSTIC CONSIDERATIONS	HISTORY	PHYSICAL EXAM

Nipple Discharge:

Presumptive cancer	Any discharge in the older patient. Itching, scaling or weeping of nipple are often present.	Breast mass and axillary node enlargement may be present. Bloody discharge may be present.
Other	Children near puberty may note minimal clear or white discharge. Patients taking phenothiazines or those suffering from neurological disease may note discharge.	Normal except for clear or white discharge.

Reference: Harrison's Principles of Internal Medicine. Seventh
Edition. Pages 582 - 587.

HISTORY

Descriptors:

General descriptors: refer to inside cover.
Onset: precise description of onset.
Aggravating factors: dusts; chest trauma; recumbent position; exertion (quantitate the amount of exertion required to precipitate dyspnea); foreign body aspiration; prolonged inactivity; recent surgery.
Relieving factors: medication (e.g. bronchodilators); upright position.
Past treatment or evaluation: ask specifically about chest x-rays, electrocardiograms, pulmonary function tests, allergic skin tests.

Associated Symptoms:

Anxiety; confusion; sense of lightheadedness; lethargy; fever or chills; night sweats; blueness or numbness of lips or fingers; cough; sputum production (color, how much, any change from usual); hemoptysis; wheezing; noisy breathing; edema; weight change; orthopnea.

Medical History:

Cigarette smoking (packs/day and duration); chronic lung disease (bronchitis; emphysema; fibrosis); heart disease; hypertension; obesity; pneumonia; chest surgery; anemia; tuberculosis.

Medications:

Bronchodilators; digitalis; diuretics; anti-hypertensive therapy; oral contraceptives.

Family History:

Breathing trouble; asthma; emphysema; tuberculosis.

Environmental History:

Where has patient lived (city, state, duration); work history (ask specifically about sandblasting, stone carving, mining, shipyards, paper mills, paint exposure, foundry and quarry work.)

PHYSICAL EXAMINATION

Measure: temperature (rectal temperatures are more accurate in patients with tachypnea); pulse; respiration rate; blood pressure; weight.

Neck: distention of neck veins at 90 degrees; tracheal shift from midline.

Chest: chest respiratory movement; tenderness to percussion (fist); dullness or hyperresonance; diaphragm movement; changes in breath sounds; rales; rhonchi; wheezes; friction rubs; egophony.

Heart: parasternal heave; apical impulse prolonged or enlarged; splitting of S_2; intensity of pulmonic component of S_2; gallops; murmurs.

Abdomen: enlarged or tender liver.

Extremities: clubbing; edema; cyanosis of nail beds.

Skin: cyanosis.

DIAGNOSTIC CONSIDERATIONS	HISTORY	PHYSICAL EXAM
Acute onset:		
Asthma (see ASTHMA)	Episodic dyspnea; known precipitants (e.g. animals, pollen, upper respiratory infection); wheezing and cough.	Respiratory distress; diffuse hyperresonance; wheezes and rhonchi; prolonged expiration.
Foreign body aspiration (airway obstruction)	Usual onset while eating in the debilitated, inebriated or semiconscious patient.	Complete Obstruction: severe respiratory distress manifested by cyanosis, gasping and loss of consciousness unless object is immediately removed from the throat. Incomplete Obstruction: Tachypnea; stridor; localized wheezing and decrease of breath sounds.
Hyperventilation	Acute onset; very anxious patient; associated with perioral and extremity paresthesia,	Normal exam between attacks. Marked tachypnea with deep sighing respirations; normal temperature; normal

DIAGNOSTIC CONSIDERATIONS	HISTORY	PHYSICAL EXAM
Acute onset:		
Hyperventilation (continued)	sense of light-headedness. Poorly described chest discomfort.	chest exam. Signs/symptoms reproduced by hyperventilation and aborted by rebreathing into paper bag.
Pneumonia	Onset over hours or days; usually coupled with sputum (green/yellow) production; fever or shaking, chills; occasional hemoptysis; pleuritic chest pain.	Tachypnea; fever usually over 101°; asymmetric chest expansion; localized dullness with increased breath sounds; rales, wheezes (local or generalized) purulent sputum.
Pneumothorax	Sudden onset of dyspnea, usually with pleuritic pain; may occur spontaneously, following chest trauma or in persons with asthma or obstructive lung disease.	Unilateral hyperresonance to percussion, decreased chest movement, and breath sounds on the same side; trachea may be deviated to opposite side.
Pulmonary edema	Severe dyspnea; precipitous onset; worse when recumbent; sputum often produced (frothy).	Patient sits up and gasps for breath; tachypnea; bilateral moist rales over lower ½ lungs; wheezes; neck vein distention at 90 degrees; gallop rhythm; cool moist skin.
Pulmonary infarction/emboli	Massive emboli may cause the sudden onset of dyspnea, dull chest pain, apprehension, sweating and faintness. Less massive emboli or infarction may cause pleuritic chest pain, cough and hemoptysis.	Tachypnea, tachycardia; increased pulmonic component of second heart sound; rales; S_3 or S_4. A pleural friction rub may be present. The physical examination is often normal if the emboli or infarction are not massive.

DIAGNOSTIC CONSIDERATIONS	HISTORY	PHYSICAL EXAM
Acute onset:		
Pulmonary infarction/ emboli (continued)	Often a history of phlebitis, calf pain or immobilization of the legs is present.	Calf tenderness or swelling may be present.
Respiratory failure	Confusion; lethargy; somnolence in patient with history of chronic pulmonary disease; patient may not complain of dyspnea.	Shallow, rapid respiration with decreased breath sounds; cyanosis, obtundation; signs of pneumonia may be present.
Subacute onset:		
Anemia	May be associated with history of bleeding, easy fatigue, postural dizziness.	Pallor; tachycardia; occasional postural blood pressure drop; stool may be positive for blood.
Lung Tumor	Change in cough pattern. Hemoptysis and chest ache may occur. Patient is usually a cigarette smoker.	Usually normal. Enlarged supraclavicular nodes may be palpated.
Tuberculosis	Fever; night sweats; weight loss; chronic cough and occasional hemoptysis. Some patients note a recent exposure to active tuberculosis or a history of a positive tuberculin test.	Examination is usually normal; apical rales, weight loss, and fever may be present.

DIAGNOSTIC CONSIDERATIONS	HISTORY	PHYSICAL EXAM
Chronic:		
Chronic congestive heart failure	Dyspnea on exertion; insidious onset with acute exacerbations; associated with history of heart disease or hypertension; orthopnea; nocturnal dyspnea. The patient is often taking digitalis and diuretics.	Rales bilaterally; elevated neck veins; enlarged heart with S_3 gallop; hepatomegaly; dependent pitting edema; weight gain often present.
Chronic pulmonary disease	Dyspnea; cough and sputum production tend to be worse after arising from sleep. Patient is usually a heavy smoker or has chronic exposure to industrial dusts.	Hyperresonant lung fields; distant breath sounds; scattered rhonchi or wheezes; prolonged expiration.
Obesity	Symptoms proportional to weight; only on exertion; no history of heart or lung disease.	Obese patients with normal physical exam.

Reference: Harrison's Principles of Internal Medicine. Seventh
           Edition. Pages 166 - 170.

HISTORY

Descriptors:

General descriptors: refer to inside cover.
Onset: precisely define type of onset and duration; specify the child's age.
Aggravating factors: dust; trauma; exertion (quantitate the amount of exertion required to precipitate dyspnea); foreign body inhalation.
Past treatment or evaluation: ask specifically about chest x-rays.

Associated Symptoms:
Anxiety; change in voice; drooling; sore throat; trouble swallowing; decreased eating; cough; sputum production (color, how much); wheezing; blueness of lips or fingers; fever or chills; weight loss.

Medical History:
Asthma; lung or heart disease; cystic fibrosis; past pneumonias; T.B.; Measles or other infectious disease in past 2 weeks.

Medications:
Any.

Family History:
T.B.; asthma; cystic fibrosis; others in family with a recent "cold" or cough.

False Positive Considerations:
The normal young infant may have "rattling" noisy breathing until his upper airways enlarge sufficiently (up to age 3-5 months).

PHYSICAL EXAMINATION

Measure: temperature (rectal); pulse; respiration rate; weight. Note if grunting respiration.
Nose: flaring nostrils.
Throat: (do not use instrument examination in child with drooling and severe stridor); erythema; swollen tonsils.
Chest: movement; symmetry; dullness or hyperresonance; change in breath sounds; rales; rhonchi; wheezes; lower rib retraction.
Heart: murmurs, rubs; gallops.
Extremities: clubbing.
Skin: cyanosis.

GENERAL CONSIDERATIONS

Usual <u>resting</u> pulse and respiratory rate of children:

Age	Pulse	(range)	Respiration	(range)
year 1	120	(80-160)	30	(25-35)
year 2	110	(80-130)	25	(20-30)
year 3	100	(80-130)	25	(20-30)
year 8	90	(70-110)	20	(18-25)

DIAGNOSTIC CONSIDERATIONS	HISTORY	PHYSICAL EXAM
Acute/subacute:		
Asthma (intrinsic, allergic)	Episodic, often with known precipitants, but wheezing is noted between attacks of dyspnea; usually does not occur in children under 5 years.	Respiratory distress; diffuse hyperresonance; wheezes, rhonchi and decreased breath sounds; prolonged expiration.
Bronchiolitis	Usually noted in children under 6 months of age. Usually does not respond to bronchodilator therapy.	Fever; marked tachypnea; flaring nostrils; rib retractions; prolonged expiration; decreased breath sounds. Eventual cyanosis, wheezes and rales may be present.
Croup (laryngotracheobronchitis)	Child usually 6 months to 3 years of age; onset following several days of "cold"; eventual barking cough, wheezing, hoarseness, and difficulty with air movement.	Minimal fever; lower rib retraction with respiration; inspiratory or expiratory wheezes.

DIAGNOSTIC CONSIDERATIONS	HISTORY	PHYSICAL EXAM
Acute/subacute:		
Epiglottitis	Children aged 3-7; acute stridor; muffled speaking; sore throat; trouble swallowing; drooling; extreme air hunger.	Aphonia; stridor; fever; lower rib retraction; cyanosis; drooling; red epiglottis may be present.
Foreign body	Child may suddenly gag, gasp or cough when foreign body is inhaled. Often the foreign body inhalation is not noted by the parents.	<u>Complete Obstruction:</u> severe respiratory distress manifested by cyanosis, gasping and loss of consciousness unless object is immediately removed from the throat. <u>Incomplete Obstruction:</u> Tachypnea; stridor; localized wheezing and decrease of breath sounds.
Hyperventilation	Acute onset; very anxious child usually over 6 years of age. Often associated with perioral paresthesia, light headedness, numbness in hands. May be evidence for anxiety-causing events.	Normal exam between attacks. Tachypnea; normal temperature; normal chest exam. Signs reproduced by hyperventilation and aborted by breathing into paper bag.
Pneumonia	Onset over hours or days; often yellow or green sputum; fever; sputum may be difficult to obtain from children.	High fever; tachypnea; lower rib retraction. Localized rales; dullness and increased bronchial sounds are often present.

DIAGNOSTIC CONSIDERATIONS	HISTORY	PHYSICAL EXAM
Acute/subacute:		
Pneumo-thorax	Sudden onset; usually spontaneous but may follow trauma; more common in patients with asthma. Pneumo-thorax may be seen in newborns several hours after birth.	Unilateral hyperreso-nance, decreased chest movement and breath sounds. If severe, tracheal shift to opposite side is pre-sent.
Chronic/recurrent:		
Asthma: SEE ABOVE		
Chronic heart or respira-tory dis-ease	Undeveloped child; often cyanosis; attacks of short-ness of breath, squatting; marked-ly abnormal exercise tolerance all the time. Feeding de-creased in the newborn.	Tachypnea; tachycardia; cyanosis; murmurs; clubbing commonly noted.
Other: (foreign body; seg-mental lung collapse; fibrocystic disease; chronic in-fections, particularly tuberculosis).	Cough; weight loss; recurrent foul spu-tum; recurrent pulmonary infections. Exposure to Tuber-culosis may be present.	Weight loss; localized lung abnormalities may be present on chest examination, but often normal chest exam.

HISTORY

Descriptors:

General descriptors: refer to inside cover.
Was there excessive or prolonged bleeding at the time of birth (from the umbilicus), past tooth extractions, surgery or following lacerations.

Associated Symptoms:

Fever; chills; headache; swollen lymph nodes; joint swelling; dark or bloody urine; black, tarry bowel movements; jaundice, skin rashes, or infections.

Medical History:

Liver disease; valvular heart disease; hemophilia; lupus erythematosis.

Medications:

Adrenal steroids; diuretics; warfarin (Coumadin); any others.

Family History:

Hemophilia; bleeding or bruising tendency.

PHYSICAL EXAMINATION

Measure: temperature.
Heart: murmurs.
Abdomen: enlarged liver or spleen.
Extremities: check joints for swelling.
Skin: jaundice; location and description of any lesions, bruises or petechiae.
Nodes: enlargement.

GENERAL CONSIDERATIONS

"Easy bruising" which is common to all true bleeding disorders is a very common complaint in persons who have no obvious disease and have noticed "easy bruising" for years. This type of apparently benign disorder is often seen in older patients. True bleeding disorders are characterized by prolonged bleeding from lacerations, tooth extractions, and by spontaneous bleeding.

GENERAL CONSIDERATIONS

True bleeding disorders can be classified into two distinct
categories which are each associated with certain types of
underlying diseases.

Bleeding disorders caused by lack or dysfunction of coagula-
tion factors are usually manifested by large superficial
bruises and spontaneous bleeding into joints and deep tissues.
Such bleeding is usually due to hereditary disease (hemophilia),
warfarin (Coumadin) anticoagulents and severe liver disease.

Bleeding disorders caused by lack or dysfunction of platelets
or fragility of blood vessels are usually manifested by small superficial bruises and petechiae and prolonged bleeding. A reduction
in the platelet count may be caused by drugs (e.g. diuretics),
diseases such as leukemia, allergic vascular disease of children
(Henoch-Schonlein), inflammatory vascular diseases (Systemic
Lupus Erythematosis) and certain infections (bacterial endocarditis, Rocky Mountain spotted fever, disseminated meningococcus). Adrenal steroid medications in pharmacological doses,
rare hereditary diseases, and some of the diseases affecting
platelets listed above may also cause increased bruising by
weakening blood vessel walls.

Reference: Harrison's Principles of Internal Medicine.   Seventh
             Edition.   Pages 300 - 308.

HISTORY

Descriptors:

General descriptors: refer to inside cover.
Location/Character:
  Electrical: point of contact; source of electricity
    (estimates of the power of the source; i.e., volts or
    amperes).
  Flame: was the face burned.
  Chemical: type of chemical; was contact on face or in
    eyes; was chemical swallowed.

Associated Symptoms:

Pain; blistering; dyspnea; loss of consciousness.

Medications:

Last tetanus shot; total number of tetanus shots.

PHYSICAL EXAMINATION

Measure: lying and sitting blood pressure and pulse; respirations.
Skin: estimate percent of burn and depth by testing sensation
  with pin in burned areas.

GENERAL CONSIDERATIONS

The extent of burned skin must be estimated to guide replacement of body fluids lost through the skin. Burns to the face
are particularly worrisome because severe respiratory damage
is possible. Electrical burns require special consideration
because severe tissue damage may be hidden under seemingly
normal skin. The presence of chemical skin burns, particularly
in children, may direct attention from the fact that the child
actually ingested the chemical.

DIAGNOSTIC CONSIDERATIONS	HISTORY	PHYSICAL EXAM
Depth of burn		
1st degree	Painful	Pinprick sense intact; red, dry skin.

DIAGNOSTIC CONSIDERATIONS	HISTORY	PHYSICAL EXAM

Depth of burn

2nd degree	Mostly painful.	Pinprick sense often intact; blisters with underlying red moist tissue.
3rd degree	No pain.	Skin is charred or leathery; may be white under surface; no pinprick sensation.

HISTORY

Descriptors:

General descriptors: refer to inside cover.
Onset: was it related to chest trauma. Is the onset of pain predictable.
Aggravating factors: emotional upset; swallowing; cold weather; sexual intercourse; deep breathing; coughing; neck, arm or chest movement; position change.
Relieving factors: food; antacids; nitroglycerin; resting; change of position; massage of painful area. How quickly is relief obtained.
Past treatment or evaluation: electrocardiogram; upper gastrointestinal X-ray; chest X-ray.

Associated Symptoms:

Anxiety; depression; faintness; palpitation; numbness or tingling in hands or around mouth; fever; shaking chills; sweating; syncope; cough; sputum production; hemoptysis; dyspnea; tenderness; trouble swallowing; nausea; vomiting; leg swelling or pain; weight change.

Medical History:

Lung disease; asthma; chest surgery; chest injury; cardiovascular disease; high blood pressure; diabetes; elevated cholesterol or triglyceride; angina; phlebitis; emotional problems.

Medications:

Oral contraceptives; diuretics; digitalis; bronchodilators; nitroglycerin ; tranquilizers; sedatives; antacids.

Family History:

Cardiovascular disease (particularly with premature death); diabetes; high blood pressure; elevated blood lipids.

Environmental History:

Cigarette smoking. Is patient pregnant.

PHYSICAL EXAMINATION

Measure: blood pressure; pulse in both arms; respiratory rate; weight; temperature.
Chest: rales; friction rub; change in breath sounds or percussion note; tenderness of chest wall.
Heart: gallops; murmurs; pericardial rubs.
Extremities: leg edema; swelling, warmth or tenderness; redness; venous prominence in calf or thigh.

GENERAL CONSIDERATIONS

Chest pains that are aggravated by chest movement or deep breathing are generally musculoskeletal or pleuritic/Pericarditic in origin. Other types of chest pain are usually due to cardio-vascular pulmonary or gastrointestinal disease. The diagnostic considerations listed below follow these general subdivisions of chest pain.

DIAGNOSTIC CONSIDERATIONS	HISTORY	PHYSICAL EXAM
Musculoskeletal Causes		
Chest wall ache	Often noted to be worse with movement or deep breathing; there may be a history of trauma to the involved area or violent coughing spells.	Chest wall tenderness often noted.
Rib fracture	History of chest trauma.	Point tenderness over ribs often with under-lying crepitation.
Neck pain referred to chest.	Pain worsened with neck movement.	Pressure over neck or movement of neck may produce upper chest or arm aching.
Arthritis/ Bursitis	May follow pro-longed coughing.	Tenderness over shoulder or rib joints (especially sterno-costal joints); tenderness of muscles often at lower chest margin.

DIAGNOSTIC CONSIDERATIONS	HISTORY	PHYSICAL EXAM
Pleuritis/ Pericarditis (Secondary to infection, or inflammation of the outer surface of the heart or lungs).	Pain is sharp and aggravated by deep breathing or coughing; pleuritic pain can be anywhere in chest; pericardial pain is usually precordial or retrosternal.	A pericardial or pleural friction rub is often heard. Localized rales, alterations in breath sounds or percussion note may be present in some diseases causing pleuritic pain.
Secondary to Cardiovascular Disease	Patients with hypertension, diabetes and elevated serum cholesterol or triglycerides are particularly prone to develop cardiovascular disease.	
Myocardial infarction	Severe, often crushing, retrosternal pain with nausea and vomiting and diaphoresis. Pain not relieved by nitroglycerin and lasts an hour or longer.	Patient may be pale and sweaty; cardiac exam may reveal arrhythmia, murmurs or gallop rhythm.
Classic angina pectoris	Retrosternal chest pain brought on by exertion; relieved by rest; pain may radiate to the left arm. Nitroglycerin characteristically relieves the pain within 2-3 minutes.	An S_3 heard only during an attack is diagnostic; an S_4 is often present between attacks.
Pre-infarction angina (or crescendo angina)	Attacks of classic angina that are increasingly easily provoked; more frequent and/or severe. Nitroglycerin may have progressively less effect on pain.	An S_3 heard only during an attack is diagnostic; an S_4 is often present between attacks.

DIAGNOSTIC CONSIDERATIONS	HISTORY	PHYSICAL EXAM
Secondary to Cardiovascular Disease		
Dissecting thoracic aortic aneurysm	Ripping, tearing chest pain which is maximal at onset and may even be described as pulsatile; may start between scapulae; syncope may occur. History of hypertension or associated abdominal pain may be present.	Carotid, radial or femoral pulses may be unequal or absent; murmur of aortic insufficiency may be heard; hypertension often present.
Secondary to Pulmonary Disease		
Pneumo-thorax	Acute onset of pleuritic pain and dyspnea; often seen in young adults or patients with asthma or chronic obstructive lung disease.	Unilateral hyper-resonance to percussion, diminished breath sounds and chest expansion on the same side; trachea may be deviated to opposite side.
Pulmonary embolus	Massive emboli may cause the sudden onset of dyspnea, dull chest pain, apprehension, sweating and faintness. Less massive emboli or infarction may cause pleuritic chest pain, cough and hemoptysis. Often a history of phlebitis, calf pain or immobilization of the legs is present.	Tachypnea, tachycardia; increased pulmonic component of second heart sound; rales; S_3 or S_4. A pleural friction rub may be present. The physical examination is often normal if the emboli or infarction are not massive. Calf tenderness or swelling may be present.

DIAGNOSTIC CONSIDERATIONS	HISTORY	PHYSICAL EXAM
Secondary to Pulmonary Disease		
Pneumonia	Onset over hours or days; usually coupled with sputum (green/yellow) production; fever or shaking, chills; occasional hemoptysis; pleuritic chest pain.	Tachypnea; fever usually over 101°; asymmetric chest expansion; localized dullness with increased breath sounds; rales, wheezes (local or generalized) purulent sputum.
Lung Tumor	Change in cough pattern. Hemoptysis and chest ache may occur. Patient is usually a cigarette smoker.	Usually normal. Enlarged supraclavicular nodes may be palpated.
Secondary to Gastrointestinal Disease		
Peptic Ulcer	Burning or gnawing, localized episodic or recurrent epigastric pain appearing 1-4 hours after meals, may be made worse by alcohol, aspirin, steroids or other anti-inflammatory medications; relieved by antacids or food.	Deep epigastric tenderness.
Cholecystitis	Colicky pain in epigastrium or right upper quadrant, occasionally radiating to right scapula; colicky with nausea, vomiting, fever; sometimes chills, jaundice, dark urine, light-colored stools (obstruction of common duct); may be recurrent.	Fever; right upper quadrant tenderness with guarding, occasional rebound; decreased bowel sounds.

DIAGNOSTIC CONSIDERATIONS	HISTORY	PHYSICAL EXAM
Secondary to Gastrointestinal Disease		
Reflux esophagitis	Burning, epigastric or substernal pain radiating up to jaws, worse when lying flat or bending over, particularly soon after meals; relieved by antacids or sitting upright.	Patient often obese; normal abdominal exam.
Esophageal spasm	Severe retrosternal pain often related to eating, relieved by nitroglycerin Dysphagia is usually present.	Normal.
Esophageal tear	Acute, severe, lower retrosternal pain, often following vomiting (Mallory-Weiss), esophageal instrumentation, or penetrating wound to neck.	Low blood pressure; sweating; pallor; a crunching crepitant sound is heard over the sternum with each heart beat (mediastinal crunch).
Esophageal stricture	Chronic, retrosternal pain or 'heartburn'. Patient may regurgitate food into throat.	Normal.
Esophageal Cancer	Chronic progressive complaints that food "sticks" or cause aching, persistent retrosternal pain.	May reveal cachexia and weight loss.

DIAGNOSTIC CONSIDERATIONS	HISTORY	PHYSICAL EXAM
Functional Chest Pain	Poorly described chest discomfort that is often transcient and associated with anxiety and hyperventilation.	Normal examination. Hyperventilation often reproduces the symptoms.

Reference: Harrison's Principles of Internal Medicine. Seventh Edition. Pages 24 - 30.

HISTORY

Descriptors:
- General descriptors: refer to inside cover.
- Onset: exactly how long has the patient appeared confused.
- Character: It is extremely important to get detailed information from someone who knows the patient well. Can the patient remember time, place, person and recent events; can the patient successfully complete simple calculations.
- Aggravating factors: head trauma; recent alcohol or drug intake or cessation of a chronic alcohol or drug habit; recent change in patient's home, job or relationships; recent medical, surgical or neurological disease.
- Past treatment or evaluation: has patient had previous neurological evaluation, particularly brain scan, lumbar tap, or electroencephalogram.

Associated Symptoms:
Change in attention span, ability to concentrate or mood; hallucinations; lethargy or stupor; excessive activity; changes in sensation or ability to move extremities; headache; fever; vomiting; breathing trouble.

Medical History:
Any chronic medical or neurological disease; recent surgery or childbirth; alcoholism and drug abuse; any history of emotional problems or psychiatric hospitalizations.

Medications:
Barbiturates; tranquilizers; antidepressants; amphetamines; LSD; mescaline; cocaine; marijuana; adrenal steroids; atropine and belladonna; alcohol.

PHYSICAL EXAMINATION

Measure: blood pressure; pulse; temperature; respiration.
Mental status: check: chronology of recent presidents; ability to recall three objects after five minutes; ability to subtract 7 from 100 and continue subtracting 7 from remainder; does patient know where he is and the month, day and year; ability to abstract from proverbs.
Eyes: check pupils for equality in size and reactivity to light. Check fundus for absent venous pulsations or papilledema.
Neck: thyroid enlargement; check for stiffness.
Chest: rales or wheezes.
Heart: murmurs, rubs or gallops.
Abdomen: liver or spleen enlargement; masses; ascites.
Rectal: check stool for occult blood.
Extremities: cyanosis or edema.
Skin: jaundice, spider angiomata.
Pulses: check strength of carotid pulses. Listen for bruit.

PHYSICAL EXAMINATION
(continued)

Neurological: check sensation to pinprick in all extremities;
strength of all extremities; deep tendon reflexes and plantar
response; cranial nerve function.
Special: check for suck and grasp reflexes. check for excessive
resistance of extremities to passive movement (paratonia).

GENERAL CONSIDERATIONS

Acute confusional states:
It is important to separate two types of acute confusional states.

The delirious person is usually overactive, grossly disoriented and actively hallucinating. Delirium is generally the
result of the sudden development or worsening of a medical,
surgical or neurological disease or an acute abstinence from
drug and alcohol intake. The delirious patient is at some
risk to injure himself or others and consequently sedatives
and tranquilizers are frequently used to help manage the
patient. Generally, however, the delirium is self-limited
and treatment is best directed at the underlying disorder.

The person who requires stimulation to stay awake is defined
as being stuporous. Stuporous patients are often confused and
disoriented, but they generally do not hallucinate and are
definitely not overactive. Since the stuporous patient is
near coma, treatment with sedatives and tranquilizers so often
helpful in managing the delirious patient could be dangerous
and cause the patient to become comatose. (See UNCONSCIOUS
for the diagnostic considerations of STUPOR and COMA).

The elderly senile patient who becomes suddenly ill and
delirious is often not very active and thus may appear stuporous.

Chronic Confusional States:

Dementia is the chronic loss of memory and intellectual function.
Questions of recent memory and ability to calculate are the
simplest clinical tests for assessing the presence of moderate
to severe dementia. Dementia usually becomes apparent in the
older person for no apparent reason (so-called senile dementias).
In all age groups underlying neurological disease (e.g. pre-
senile dementia, neurosyphillis, Huntington's chorea, subdural
hematoma, brain tumor) can cause dementia. Severely demented
patients often have primitive reflexes (suck and grasp reflexes)
and resist movement of extremities (paratonia).

GENERAL CONSIDERATIONS
(continued)

Psychosis:

The psychotic person may appear confused because of the disor-
dered illogical thoughts he may express. Generally,
however, the psychotic patient has neither impairment of intellect
nor disorientation. Although psychoses rarely result from
medications (amphetamines and adrenal steroids), most psychoses
first become apparent in young adults in whom there is no
obvious medical or neurological disease.

Reference: Harrison's Principles or Internal Medicine. Seventh
            Edition. Pages 149-156, 1871-1903.

HISTORY

Descriptors:
    General Descriptors: refer to inside cover.
    Onset: how many stools per day or week; has there been recent
        change in the character or frequency of movements.
    Past treatment or evaluation: past barium enema or proc-
        toscopic exam.

Associated Symptoms:
    Abdominal pain; blood in stools; pain with defecation;
    diarrhea alternating with hard stool; weight loss; anxiety;
    depression.

Medical History:
    Colitis; emotional problems; diverticular disease.

Medications:
    Laxatives; enemas; tranquilizers; sedatives; opiates; antacids;
    anticholinergic medications.

Environmental History:
    What does the patient normally eat.

PHYSICAL EXAMINATION

    Abdominal: masses; tenderness.
    Rectal: stool for occult blood; is the rectum full of feces
        or empty; is anus tender.

GENERAL CONSIDERATIONS

In adults the commonest causes of chronic constipation are the
laxative habit and a diet high in carbohydrate and low in fiber
content (whole grain cereals, raw vegetables).

Other major considerations include:
1. Partial bowel obstruction (tumor): recent change in bowel
habits; rarely abdominal mass is present.
2. Decreased defecation reflex: either due to habitual constipation (rectum will be full of feces) or the chronic laxative
habit.
3. Inflammation of anus: pain on defecation;anus will be tender.
4. Irritable bowel: chronic history of anxiety causing loose
stools and lower abdominal pain (often cluster in the morning)
alternating with constipation.
5. Other considerations include the side effect of opiate and
anticholinergic medications, aluminum containing antacids and

CONSTIPATION
(ADULT)
(Continued)

GENERAL CONSIDERATIONS
(Continued)

disease or weakness of the abdominal muscles.

Reference: Harrison's Principles of Internal Medicine. Seventh
Edition. Pages 217-218.

HISTORY

Descriptors:
    General descriptors: refer to inside cover
    Onset: has toilet training been recently enforced.
    Character: how many stools per day or week.

Associated Symptoms:
    Vomiting; excessive urination; crying during bowel movement;
    change in appetite; abdominal swelling; blood on stool.

Medications:
    Any.

Environmental History:
    What type of diet has the child had; recent change in diet;
    if formula is used, how is it diluted. How many bowel
    movements per day do the parents expect the child to have.

PHYSICAL EXAMINATION

    Measure: weight.
    Abdomen: masses; tenderness; distention.
    Rectal: examine for fissures (may need anoscope). Is rectum
      full of feces or empty.
    Skin: check for skin turgor.

GENERAL CONSIDERATIONS

Adults and children may normally have a bowel movement as
seldom as once or twice a week. The commonest cause for
constipation is parental concern that their child should have
a bowel movement every day.

Concern for regularity or bowel control (toilet training) can
cause a child to become so anxious about having a bowel movement that the evacuation reflex is inhibited. Rectal examination will often reveal feces in the rectum.

Other causes for constipation include the following:

DIAGNOSTIC CONSIDERATIONS	HISTORY	PHYSICAL EXAM
Rectal fissures	Pain on bowel movement; blood on stool.	Painful rectal examination; rectal fissure noted on anoscopy.

CONSTIPATION
(PEDIATRIC)
(Continued)

DIAGNOSTIC CONSIDERATIONS	HISTORY	PHYSICAL EXAM
Bowel obstruction (see also ABDOMINAL PAIN)	Abdominal distention; decreased volume or caliber of stools; obstipation; vomiting and weight loss.	Abdominal distention; masses or tenderness are often present. Rectum may be empty of stool.
Abnormal Feeding (infant)	The formula may be excessively concentrated or fluid intake may be inadequate.	Weight loss and dehydration are noted. Rectal exam is normal.

HISTORY

Descriptors:
  General descriptors: refer to inside cover
  Onset: was there head trauma.
  Location/radiation: precise description of spread of seizure
    and location of post seizure paralysis.

Associated Symptoms:
  "funny feeling" before or after attack; change in vision,
  hearing, ability to move or sensory functions; headache;
  fever or chills; stiff neck; tongue biting; loss of
  consciousness; loss of bladder or bowel control; palpitations;
  trouble breathing; nausea/vomiting.

Medical History:
  Diabetes; hypertension; alcoholism; birth trauma; previous
  meningitis, encephalitis, epilepsy; drug abuse; severe head
  trauma; chronic kidney disease; cerebrovascular accidents.

Medications:
  Alcohol; anticonvulsants; insulin; oral hypoglycemic agents;
  antihypertensives; sedatives.

Family History:
  Epilepsy.

Environmental History:
  Possibility of poison ingestion, particularly lead or insecticides.

PHYSICAL EXAMINATION

  Measure: blood pressure; pulse; temperature.
  Head: evidence of trauma.
  Eyes: pupil equality and reactivity to light. Fundus:
    absent venous pulsations, hemorrhages, or papilledema.
  Mouth: evidence of tongue biting.
  Neck: check for stiffness.
  Heart: murmurs or irregularity.
  Genital/Rectal: evidence of incontinence.
  Skin: cyanosis.
  Pulses: check strength of carotid pulses, listen for bruit.
  Neurological: sensation to pinprick in all extremities; strength
    of all extremities; deep tendon reflexes and plantar response;
    cranial nerve function.

GENERAL CONSIDERATIONS

  There are four common types of convulsive disorders:
  Grand mal seizures begin with a sudden loss of consciousness

GENERAL CONSIDERATIONS (Continued)

followed by rhythmic total body rigidity and relaxations, loss
of bowel and/or bladder function and often a brief comatose
state.

Petit mal seizures are brief "absence" attacks occuring most
commonly in prepubescent children. Loss of consciousness
extremely brief and no gross convulsive activity is present.

Focal or marching seizures begin in one area of the body. If
the convulsive activity spreads over the entire body
(Jacksonian march) it climaxes in a grand mal type of convulsion. These seizures are usually associated with demon-
strable brain pathology.

Psychomotor seizures are characterized by a feeling of anxiety
or an unusual sensation followed by an alteration in consciousness. The alteration in consciousness is associated
with complex and varied states of thinking, behavior and
feeling (i.e. lip smacking, fumbling with buttons, hallucinations).

Many of the persons suffering from convulsive diseases have
'mixed' seizures in which characteristics of any of the four
common seizures listed above occur.

Many convulsions first occur in children and adolescents who
may have a family history of epilepsy but are otherwise normal.
The cause for these convulsions is unclear (idiopathic epilepsy).

Other causes for convulsive diseases are listed below:

DIAGNOSTIC CONSIDERATIONS	HISTORY	PHYSICAL EXAM
Secondary to inherited diseases (phenylketonuria, tuberous sclerosis) or perinatal pro-blems (birth injury)	Onset of convulsions usually before 4 years of age. The child often is retarded in development.	Congenital malformations or developmental retar-dation are often present.
Secondary to:		
Cerebral trauma	Severe head injury usually causing frac-ture or penetration of the skull. Seizures may begin many months after trauma.	Localized neurological abnormalities are fre-quently present.

DIAGNOSTIC CONSIDERATIONS	HISTORY	PHYSICAL EXAM
Secondary to:		
Cerebral tumor	The older patient with no history of previous seizures; severe persistent headaches; nausea and vomiting in the later stages. Occasionally a history of other malignancy which might spread to the brain (e.g. cancer of lung or breast).	Eventually neurological abnormalities, loss of venous pulsations in the fundus, and papilledema are present.
Cerebrovascular accident	The patient is frequently over 60 years of age; sudden onset of focal paralysis	Localized neurological abnormalities; the patient may not regain consciousness.
Hypertensive encephalopathy	Hypertensive history; headache; blurred vision; stupor	Diastolic blood pressure is usually greater than 140 mm of mercury; fundi show hemorrhages and papilledema.
Infection (meningitis, encephalitis, brain abscess)	Fever; chills; headache. Patient often becomes stuporous.	Localized neurological abnormalities, stiff neck and fever may be present.
Other causes of brief, frequently non-recurrent convulsions		
Fever (Pediatric)	Children ages 6 months to 5 years; sudden elevation of temperature (20 to 30% of children with simple febrile convulsions eventually develop idopathic epilepsy).	Fever. Otherwise normal.
Alcohol Withdrawal	See ALCOHOLISM	

HISTORY

Descriptors:
    General descriptors: refer to inside cover.
    Aggravating factors: (pediatric) possibility of foreign body
      aspiration.
    Past treatment or evaluation: previous tuberculin skin test or
      chest X-ray.

Associated Symptoms:
    Runny nose; sore throat; facial pain; sputum production (note
    color and amount); hemoptysis; dyspnea; orthopnea; wheezing;
    chest pain; fever; sweats; weight loss.

Medical History:
    Past pulmonary infections; cardiovascular disease; chronic lung
    disease; tuberculosis.

Family History:
    Tuberculosis.

Environmental History:
    Cigarette smoking; chronic exposure to industrial dusts (asbestos,
    rock dust); exposure to someone with active tuberculosis;
    (pediatric) past immunization for whooping cough.

PHYSICAL EXAMINATION

    Measure: temperature; weight; respiratory rate.
    Head: sinus tenderness.
    Throat: erythema
    Chest: dullness to percussion; rales; wheezes; prolonged
      expiration.
    Heart: murmurs; gallops.

DIAGNOSITC CONSIDERATIONS	HISTORY	PHYSICAL EXAM
Adult and Pediatric **Acute**		
Upper respiratory infection (including sore throat, sinusitis)	Runny nose; sore throat; facial pain; general malaise; minimal sputum.	Chest exam usually normal. Pharyngitis and sinus tenderness may be present.

DIAGNOSITC CONSIDERATIONS	HISTORY	PHYSICAL EXAM
Bacterial and mycoplasma infections	Onset over hours or days; usually coupled with sputum (green/yellow) production; fever or chills; occasional hemoptysis; pleuritic chest pain.	Tachypnea; Fever usually over 101 degrees; asymmetric expansion; localized dullness with increased breath sounds; rales, wheezes (local or generalized); purulent sputum.

Pediatric-Acute

Croup (laryngotracheobronchitis)	Child usually 6 months to 3 years of age; onset following several days of upper respiratory infection; eventual barking cough, wheezing, hoarseness and difficulty with air movement.	Minimal fever; lower rib retraction with inspiration; inspiratory or expiratory wheezes.
Whooping Cough	As in croup. The child may be younger and unimmunized. Inspiratory whooping; nausea and vomiting may be present.	Fever, stridor and wheezing.

Pediatric-Chronic

(foreign body; segmental lung collapse; fibrocystic disease; chronic infections; particularly tuberculosis)	Chronic cough; weight loss; recurrent foul sputum; recurrent pulmonary infections; exposure to tuberculosis may be present.	Weight loss; localized lung abnormalities may be present on chest examination but often the chest is normal.

Adult-Chronic

Cigarette smoking	Minimal sputum	Usually normal but eventually leads to abnormalities described under chronic lung disease.

DIAGNOSITC CONSIDERATIONS	HISTORY	PHYSICAL EXAM
Chronic lung disease (chronic bronchitis and emphysema)	Dyspnea; cough and sputum production tend to be worse after arising from sleep. Patient is usually a heavy cigarette smoker or has had chronic exposure to industrial dusts.	Hyperresonant lung fields; distant breath sounds; scattered ronchi or wheezes; prolonged expiration.
Lung tumor	Change in cough pattern. Hemoptysis and chest ache may occur. Patient is usually a cigarette smoker.	Usually normal. Enlarged supraclavicular nodes may be palpated.
Tuberculosis	Fever, night sweats, weight loss; chronic cough and occasional hemoptysis. Some patients note a recent exposure to active tuberculosis or a history of a positive tuberculin test.	Examination is usually normal; apical rales, weight loss and fever may be present.
Congestive heart failure or mitral stenosis	Nocturnal coughing; orthopnea; dyspnea; paroxysmal nocturnal dyspnea.	Moist rales at both bases; ankle edema. Heart exam may reveal an S_3 gallop, a diastolic murmur or a loud pulmonic component of the second heart sound.

Reference: Harrison's Principles of Internal Medicine. Seventh
            Edition. Pages 196-197.

HISTORY

Descriptors:
    General descriptors: refer to inside cover
                    Amount of blood coughed up; Is coughing of
    blood a recurrent problem.
    Past treatment or evaluation: Previous chest X-ray or
      tuberculin skin test.

Associated Symptoms:
    Chest pain; dyspnea; wheezing; orthopnea; sputum production;
    fever; chills; decrease in weight; leg pain or ankle swelling.

Medical History:
    Tuberculosis; valvular heart disease; bronchitis or bron-
    chiectasis; pulmonary embolism; lung tumor.

Environmental History:
    Cigarette smoking.

False Positives:
    Vomiting blood; expectoration of blood from nasopharyngeal
    bleeding.

PHYSICAL EXAMINATION

      Measure: temperature; blood pressure; weight.
      Chest: rales; wheezing; pleural friction rub.
      Heart: murmurs; gallops.
      Extremities: calf tenderness or swelling; ankle edema.

DIAGNOSTIC CONSIDERATIONS	HISTORY	PHYSICAL EXAM
Acute-Life Threatening		
Bronchitis or Bronchiectasis	Chronic cough and dyspnea with sputum production usually worse in the mornings. Sputum production may be noted only in certain positions. Occasional hemoptysis.	Diffuse rhonchi and wheezes; prolonged expiration may be present.

DIAGNOSTIC CONSIDERATIONS	HISTORY	PHYSICAL EXAM
Pneumonia	Onset over hours or days; usually coupled with sputum (green/yellow) production; fever or chills; occasional hemoptysis; pleuritic chest pain.	Tachypnea; Fever usually over 101 degrees; asymmetric expansion; localized dullness with increased breath sounds; rales, wheezes (local or generalized); purulent sputum.
Pulmonary embolus	Massive emboli may cause the sudden onset of dyspnea, dull chest pain, apprehension, sweating and faintness. Less massive emboli or infarction may cause pleuritic chest pain, cough and hemoptysis. Often a history of phlebitis, calf pain or immobilization of the legs is present.	Tachypnea, tachycardia; increased pulmonic component of second heart sound; rales; S_3 or S_4. A pleural friction rub may be present. The physical examination is often normal if the emboli or infarction are not massive. Calf tenderness or swelling may be present.
Lung Tumor	see COUGH	
Tuberculosis	see COUGH	
Mitral stenosis	History of rheumatic fever or valvular heart disease; dyspnea; orthopnea.	Diastolic murmur; moist basilar rales; ankle edema.
Unknown (idiopathic)	Usually follows the persistent cough of an upper respiratory infection.	Chest examination is usually normal.

Reference: Harrison's Principles of Internal Medicine. Seventh
            Edition. Pages 197-199.

HISTORY

Descriptors:

General descriptors: refer to inside cover.
Onset: did cramps begin immediately after onset of menses
   (menarche) or later in life; relation of cramps to bleeding; when was the last menstrual period and was it normal.

Associated Symptoms:

Fever; shaking, chills; weight gain during menses; anxiety
or depression; nausea; vomiting; back pain; dysuria; vaginal
discharge; excessive menstrual or intermenstrual bleeding.

Medical History:

Endometriosis; malposition of uterus; pelvic inflammatory
disease; emotional problems; number of previous pregnancies.

Medications:

Diuretics; tranquilizers; oral contraceptives.

False Positive Considerations:

Pain not associated with menses.

PHYSICAL EXAMINATION

Measure: temperature.
Abdomen: masses, tenderness. Flanks - punch tenderness.
Pelvic/Rectal: check for masses, tenderness, vaginal discharge. If virginal introitus, check for imperforate
   hymen.

DIAGNOSTIC CONSIDERATIONS	HISTORY	PHYSICAL EXAM
Menstrual cramps	Recurrent pain; pattern often the same since menarche; psychic tension worsens the pain as does uterine malposition or an imperforate hymen.	Usually normal. Uterine malposition or imperforate hymen may be present.
Endometriosis	Deep dull back and pelvis pain beginning after the age of 20	Small nodular pelvic masses; localized tenderness or thickening

DIAGNOSTIC CONSIDERATIONS	HISTORY	PHYSICAL EXAM
Endometriosis (continued)	and becoming progressively worse. Endometriosis is rare in women with multiple pregnancies.	of the adnexa may be present.
Pelvic inflammatory disease	Vaginal discharge occasionally with worsening of menstrual cramps or lower abdominal pain.	Temperature may be elevated. Vaginal discharge; cervical and adnexal tenderness.
Menstrual "fluid"	Pain less prominent than "bloating" or weight gain during menses.	Normal.
Urinary tract infection	May cause pain similar to menstrual cramps; usually the patient complains of dysuria, fever, shaking chills, or back pain.	Fever and flank tenderness may be present.
"Mittelschmerz"	Intermenstrual lower abdominal pain of variable intensity lasting less than 24 hours.	Normal.

For other considerations
  See also ABDOMINAL PAIN

HISTORY

Descriptors:

General descriptors: refer to inside cover.
Onset: what was patient doing when the cyanosis was noted.
Location: what part of the body is cyanotic.
Aggravating factors: does the cyanosis worsen during exertion.

Associated Symptoms:
Confusion or change in mood or personality; convulsions; headache; lethargy; dyspnea; chest pain; cough; wheezing; sputum production; poor exercise tolerance; squatting; fainting; clubbing of fingers; weight loss.

Medical History:
Cardiac, respiratory, or blood disease.

Medications:
Digitalis; diuretics; oxygen; bronchodilators; antibiotics; sedatives; pain relievers; nitroglycerin; acetanilide (Bromoselzer); phenacetin (Emperin).

Environmental History:
Aniline dye or wax crayon ingestion.

False Positive Considerations:
Extremities exposed to cold may turn "blue" in normal adults and children. Trunk and tongue remain "pink".

PHYSICAL EXAMINATION

Measure: temperature; respiration rate; blood pressure; pulse.
Neck: check for tracheal deviation.
Chest: rales; wheezes; resonance to percussion.
Heart: murmur or gallops; prolonged ventricular thrust or enlarged heart to palpation.
Extremities: clubbing; cyanosis or edema.
Pediatric: check for retraction of ribs; flaring of nostrils; growth and development parameters.

GENERAL CONSIDERATIONS

True cyanosis - a blue-purple discoloration of the lips,

GENERAL CONSIDERATIONS

tongue, trunk and nail beds - is a reflection of poor oxygena-
tion of the blood and indicates severe heart or lung disease.

In children chronic cyanosis is typically due to congenital
heart disease and will usually be accompanied by a history
of poor growth, poor exercise tolerance or squatting. Heart
murmurs, cardiac enlargement and clubbing of the digits are
often noted on physical examination.

In adults, chronic cyanosis is most commonly caused by
severe lung disease in which unventilated parts of the lung
are perfused with unoxygenated blood; often associated with
smoking.

Acute cyanosis usually indicates life threatening cardiac
or respiratory disease and is often accompanied by tachypnea.
Severe respiratory infection with fever, cough and rales;
upper airway obstruction by a foreign body; pneumothorax
marked by tracheal deviation, unilateral hyperresonance and
decreased breath sounds are all causes of acute cyanosis in
adults and children. Cardiovascular collapse, particularly
following myocardial infarction, is another cause for acute
cyanosis in the adult. The possibility of ingestion of substances that change the composition of hemoglobin (aniline
dyes, phenacetin containing medications, nitrates, sulfona-
mides) should always be considered in the adult or child with
cyanosis and no obvious cardiac or respiratory disease.

Reference: Harrison's Principles of Internal Medicine. Seventh
            Edition. Pages 170 - 172.

HISTORY

Descriptors:

General descriptors: refer to inside cover.
        Was there abdominal, lower back or urethral trauma.
Specify color of urine; dark urine only at certain times
of day; dark urine at beginning, end, or throughout urine
stream.

Associated Symptoms:
Flank or abdominal pain; dysuria; frequency; passing gravel
in urine; fever or chills; bruising or bleeding elsewhere;
yellow conjunctivae or skin (jaundice); pale stools.

Medical History:
Kidney stones; kidney disease; prostate disease; liver disease; blood disease; sickle cell disease.

Medications:
Warfarin (Coumadin); urinary analgesics (e.g. Azo Gantrisin).

Family History:
Anemias; blood diseases.

False Positive Considerations:
Prior intake of beets may cause the urine to become red. After
low fluid intake or during fever urine may become dark yellow.
Certain urinary analgesics may cause darkening of the urine.

PHYSICAL EXAMINATION

Measure: oral temperature; blood pressure.
Abdomen: Flanks - punch tenderness. Abdominal masses or
  tenderness.
Rectal: (males) - prostate enlargement.
Skin: jaundice; petechiae; ecchymoses.

GENERAL CONSIDERATIONS

The most common cause for dark urine in the adult is blood
in the urine (hematuria). Dehydration, beet and drug ingestion,
and liver disease are less common causes of dark urine.

GENERAL CONSIDERATIONS

   When patients note dysuria, abdominal or flank pain or a
change in urinary habits hematuria is usually due to cystitis,
urethritis, renal stones or renal trauma. (See URINE TROU-
BLE).

   Hematuria associated with no patient discomfort is often
secondary to renal or bladder tumor, chronic renal disease,
benign prostatic hypertrophy, hemolytic disease or generalized bleeding abnormalities. Evaluation of this 'painless'
hematuria often involves specific laboratory tests and x-ray
procedures.

Reference: Harrison's Principles of Internal Medicine. Seventh
            Edition. Pages 244 - 246.

HISTORY

Descriptors:

General descriptors: refer to inside cover.
Feeling blue, chronic complaints without organic cause, nervous.
What, if any, are known precipitating events; "do you think your illness is psychological?"; are there suicidal thoughts or plans.

Associated Symptoms:

Loss of appetite; change in sleep or sex pattern; change in bowel habits, weight, menstrual periods; forgetfulness; "funny feelings" (specify) or unusual thoughts (obsessions, fears); crying frequently; palpitations; excessive sweating; tingling of lips or fingers.

Medical History:

Psychiatric illness; alcoholism; drug abuse; any chronic disease; past suicide attempts.

Medications:

Birth control pills; methyldopa; steroids; reserpine; anti-depressants; sedatives; tranquilizers; thyroid pills; amphetamines.

Family History:

Mental illness; suicide.

Environmental:

Change in job; family finances; deaths; losses.

PHYSICAL EXAMINATION

Mental status: does the patient know where he is and the month, day and year; ability to abstract proverbs and recall the chronology of recent presidents.

GENERAL CONSIDERATIONS

Many patients have a life-long problem with anxiety. Under
certain stresses they suffer more acutely and may complain of
the physical manifestation of anxiety (sweating, palpitations,
paresthesias, trouble sleeping). In other patients severe
anxiety may appear suddenly in reaction to stress or may indicate an underlying depression or a psychosis.

When approaching the depressed or anxious patient one should
always consider the following:

First, what are the possible causes of the emotional stress:
marital, sexual, job-related problems; deaths; recent illness;
drug use (birth control pills, methyl-dopa (Aldomet), reserpine,
steroids, thyroid pills, amphetamines).

Second, how severe is the anxiety or depression. The patient's
mood must be assessed and the "biological" signs of depression
noted: loss of appetite, weight loss, sleep disturbance, loss
of sex drive, forgetfulness. If the patient is depressed,
suicidal thoughts should be investigated (see SUICIDE THOUGHTS).

Finally, features suggesting a psychosis should be noted: dis-
turbed thinking, delusions, hallucinations (see CONFUSION).

Reference: Harrison's Principles of Internal Medicine. Seventh
          Edition. Pages 1878, 1887-1895.

HISTORY

Descriptors:

General descriptors: refer to inside cover.
Onset: age at onset.
Past treatment or evaluation: how documented (blood, urine
   tests); how does patient follow disease; results of testing
   urine at home and how does patient vary his medication and
   diet.

Associated Symptoms:

Periods of weakness, nervousness, hunger or confusion; chest
discomfort; trouble breathing; change in vision; recurrent
infections; skin, leg ulcers; motor or sensory changes;
thirst; polyuria; fever.

Medical History:

Neurological disease; sensory change; kidney disease; urinary
tract infections; hypoglycemic spells (insulin "reactions");
past ketoacidosis, coma; obesity; cardiovascular disease.

Medications:

Insulin (type and number of units); oral hypoglycemics
(specify); diet (calories); diuretics.

Family History:

Diabetes.

PHYSICAL EXAMINATION

Measure: blood pressure, pulse, temperature.
Eyes: fundi for hemorrhages, exudates, new vessels; visual
   acuity.
Heart: murmurs, rubs or gallops.
Extremities: condition of feet, checking carefully for early
   ulceration -- particularly between toes.
Pulses: check all pulses.
Neurological: check sensation in feet.

GENERAL CONSIDERATIONS

The examiner should determine how the patient's diabetes has
been controlled in the past (diet, pills and/or insulin) and
how good the control has been recently (results of urine tests).

A diabetic may encounter acute problems when his blood sugar
becomes either too high or too low. Insufficient insulin or
intercurrent stress (such as infection) may lead to elevated
blood sugars and eventually to ketoacidosis marked by thirst,
excess urination and finally coma. A reduction of blood sugar
can be produced by excess insulin or other hypoglycemic agents
and by excess exertion. Patients with hypoglycemia may note
sweating, weakness, hunger and even loss of consciousness.

Diabetics are also prone to develop a number of chronic problems including infections, especially of the skin and urinary
tract, renal disease, cardiovascular disease, neurological and
ocular disorders.

Reference: Harrison's Principles of Internal Medicine.   Seventh
           Edition. Pages 532-550.

HISTORY

Descriptors:
  General descriptors: refer to inside cover.

Medications:
  Any.

Environmental:
  Cloth or disposable diapers; frequency of change; soaps used;
  baths per week; powder or creams used.

PHYSICAL EXAMINATION

Skin: pustular, scaling border, satellite lesions, crusts.

GENERAL CONSIDERATIONS

Diaper rash is an inflammation of the skin caused by contact
with substances in the urine or feces. Diaper rash is aggravated by waterproof coverings of diapers, prolonged contact
with soiled diapers and the use of ointments or creams which
might sensitize the skin.

Candida superinfection of diaper rash requires special treatment. Its presence is suggested by a scaling border of the
rash and separate satellite lesions.

A superficial vesicular rash which often becomes confluent
and produces a honey colored crust is characteristic of
impetigo and   also requires special treatment. Impetigo
is contagious.

HISTORY

Descriptors:
   General descriptors: refer to inside cover.
   Character: what is the color of the stained diaper.
   Aggravating factor: staining related to bowel movement
      or urination.

Associated Symptoms:
   Does the baby cry during passage of bowel or urine; diaper
   rash; urethral discharge; nausea; vomiting; diarrhea; fever.

Medications:
   Any.

Environmental:
   Recent change in diet that might account for staining.

PHYSICAL EXAMINATION

   Abdomen: perineal area for rash; urethral discharge or
      rectal discharge.
   Rectal: check for rectal fissure or fistula; check stool for
      occult blood.

GENERAL CONSIDERATIONS

   One must determine if the cause for the diaper staining
   is secondary to diet change or if the staining indicates
   that dark urine or blood in stools is present (see DARK
   URINE or BLOOD IN STOOLS if applicable).

   Urine colors:
      Red -- beets, blood, amorphous urates, myoglobin,
            drugs (Diphenylhydantoin).
      Green -- bile, concentrated urine, drugs.
      Other -- usually drug related.

GENERAL CONSIDERATIONS
(Continued)

      Stool colors:
       Black -- melena, meconium, iron, bismuth.
       Green -- breast feeding, infectious diarrhea.
       Red -- blood.
       Extremely pale -- obstructive jaundice, steatorrhea,
                        antacids.

HISTORY

Descriptors:

General descriptors: refer to inside cover.
Duration; number of stools per hour or day; approximate
volume of stool; ability of patient to eat and drink without vomiting; eating of dairy or meat products within 72 hours
of onset (If yes, were such foods eaten within 6 hours of
onset).

Associated Symptoms:
Weight loss; faintness upon arising suddenly; nausea, vomiting, fever, chills; abdominal pain; blood, mucous or pus in
stool; malaise, myalgia, arthralgia, upper respiratory
illness.

Medications:
Antibiotics; any medication.

Environmental History:
Are the patient's toilet facilities shared with others; do
other people have the same problem; any people with the same
problem who ate the same food as patient. Recent or present
travel to tropical or subtropical country (If yes, do (*)
starred data base also).

PHYSICAL EXAMINATION

Measure: temperature; pulse; blood pressure; weight.
Throat: mucous membranes.
Abdomen: tenderness.
Rectal: examine stool for occult blood and pus.
Skin: turgor.
Special: gram stain stool to look for fecal polymorphonuclear
leukocytes; giardia lamblia.

*Additional Data (for Tropics or Subtropics)

History: has skin been in contact with potentially contaminated water.
Other exam: examination of fresh, warm stool for trophozoites
of Entameba Histolytica or ova of Schistosoma Mansoni.

DIAGNOSTIC CONSIDERATIONS	RELEVANT DATA BASE	INCIDENCE	COURSE
Viral - Nonbacterial	Seldom pus, blood or mucous; vomiting often present; prodrome of malaise; fever variably present; polymorpho-nuclear leukocytes are seldom present on gram stain of stool; associated upper respiratory illness common.	Common	2-3 days
Bacterial (Salmonella, Shigella, E. Coli)	Onset 24-72 hours after eating food that made others sick; pus and mu-cous often in stool; low grade fever present usually; poly-morphonuclear leuko-cytes often present on gram stain of stool.	Moderate	Days
Bacterial Toxins (staphylo-cocci, Clostridia)	Onset usually within 1-6 hours of eating food (Especially milk products or meats) that made others sick; no prodrome; no fever; severe nausea and vomiting.	Moderate	12-36 hours
Giardiasis	Acute to subacute diarrhea with bulky stools; occasional abdominal discom-fort and weight loss. Trophozoites in stool.	Common.	Days to weeks.

DIAGNOSTIC CONSIDERATIONS	RELEVANT DATA BASE	INCIDENCE	COURSE
*Schistosomal dysentery (S. Mansoni) (S. Japonicum)	Contact of skin with fecally contaminated water; Early: non-specific diarrhea, no ova in stool. Late: high fever, chills, cough, urticaria, lymphadenopathy, enlarged tender liver, ova in stool.	Common	Early: 1-2 weeks Late: Up to 3 months.
*Amebic Dysentery	History of recurrent diarrhea; fever usually not present except in severely ill patients; profuse bloody diarrhea with tenesmus; hepatomegaly and abdominal tenderness; trophozoites in stool.	Common.	Variable
*Malaria (P. falciparum, pernicious syndrome)	Cold clammy skin; hypotension; profound weakness, fainting; tender hepatomegaly; jaundice; melena; splenomegaly invariably present.	Uncommon manifestation of Malaria.	Days
*Cholera	Low blood pressure; faint pulse; poor skin turgor; sunken eyeballs; cyanosis.	Rare in Western Hemisphere; Common in epidemics.	2-7 days

DIAGNOSTIC CONSIDERATIONS	RELEVANT DATA BASE	INCIDENCE	COURSE
*Turista (travelers diarrhea)	Visitor to tropics or subtropics; stools may contain blood and leukocytes.	Common	1-2 days

* Occur principally in persons who live in tropical or subtropical countries.

Reference: Harrison's Principles of Internal Medicine. Seventh Edition. Pages 215 - 217, 855, 1021.

HISTORY

Descriptors:

General descriptors: refer to inside cover.
Character: quantitate exactly the number of bowel movements and their size each day; any bowel movements at
  night; any blood, pus or mucous in stool; color; odor.
Aggravating factors: bowel movements made worse by anxiety.
Past treatment or evaluation: past barium enema, proctoscopic
  or upper gastrointestinal xray examination.

Associated Symptoms:

Change in weight; fever or chills; skin rashes; joint or
back pain; abdominal pain (localize exactly any associated
pain); anxiety-depression; nausea; vomiting; change in bowel
habits; perirectal tenderness; rectal urgency.

Medical History:

Ankylosing spondylitis; emotional problems; diverticulosis;
known ulcerative colitis or regional enteritis; perirectal
abscess; past gastrointestinal surgery; pancreatitis; anemia;
diabetes; recurrent respiratory infections (Pediatric).

Medications:

Adrenal steroids; sedatives; tranquilizers; quinidine;
colchicine; Azulfidine; antibiotics (ampicillin or tetracycline); antispasmodics (Lomotil); laxatives; antacid
(Maalox).

Family History:

Cystic fibrosis (Pediatric).

Environmental History:

Excessive cereals, prunes and roughage may increase the bulk or
frequency of bowel movements.
Pediatric: has there been a change in milk ingestion. What
  is the nature of the diet.

PHYSICAL EXAMINATION

Measure: temperature; weight; blood pressure lying and
  standing.
Abdomen: masses; tenderness; bowel sounds.
Rectal: check for fecal impaction; stool for occult blood.
Special: gross and microscopic of stool for ova and para-
  sites.

PHYSICAL EXAMINATION

* Additional Data: (for Tropics and Subtropics)
    History: ask about cough, urticaria, skin rash; repeated
      exposure to contaminated water.

GENERAL CONSIDERATIONS

Diarrhea is defined as the frequent passage of poorly formed
stools. Most patients can easily recognize and accurately
define acute diarrhea as an abrupt change in their bowel habits.
Chronic or recurrent 'diarrhea' is often more difficult for
the patient to define since 'diarrhea' may mean malabsorption,
tenesmus or true diarrhea.

The examiner should try to distinguish whether:

1. the stools are frequent, voluminous and poorly formed
(suggestive of diarrhea).

2. the stools are large, oily, malodorous but somewhat
formed (suggestive of malabsorption).

3. the stools are frequent, formed, small, but associated
with an increased urge to defecate (tenesmus).

DIAGNOSTIC CONSIDERATIONS	RELEVANT DATA BASE	COURSE
Irritable bowel	Recurrent abdominal discomfort and/or change in bowel habits aggravated by anxiety; diarrhea often alternates with constipation; rectal urgency and mucous.	Days; recurrent
Inflammatory bowel disease (Crohns disease, ulcerative colitis)	Nocturnal diarrhea and pain; occasional blood or pus in bowel movements; abdominal pain; weight loss; anemia; joint pains; rectal fistula; fever; skin lesions.	Weeks; recurrent

DIAGNOSTIC CONSIDERATIONS	RELEVANT DATA BASE	COURSE
Adult malabsorption (secondary to bowel surgery, pancreatitis)	Large, foul smelling, light colored, oily stools; weight loss; weakness.	Years.
Pediatric Malabsorption		
Cystic Fibrosis	As in adult malabsorption; there is often a history of frequent respiratory infections or a family history of cystic fibrosis.	Variable.
Celiac Disease (gluten sensitivity)	As in adult malabsorption; weight loss may be marked. Onset usually after 6 months of age when cereals are first fed to the child.	Sensitivity to gluten usually persists for years.
Cow's milk protein allergy	Vomiting, chronic bloody diarrhea. Severe weight loss may occur.	Years.
Disaccharidase Deficiency	Watery, explosive, frothy diarrhea with a pH less than 5.5. Onset occurs soon after birth.	Variable.

DIAGNOSTIC CONSIDERATIONS	RELEVANT DATA BASE	COURSE
Drug induced	Ampicillin, tetracycline, laxatives; Maalox; para-amino salicyclic acid, phenothiazine tranquilizers, colchicine, quinidine.	Weeks-months.
Secondary to partial obstruction by tumor or fecal impaction	Abdominal mass, rectal mass or fecal impaction.	Variable.
Secondary to diabetes	Often a long history of diabetes usually associated with neurological dysfunction.	Variable.
Giardiasis	Malodorous stools and weight loss; trophozoites in stool.	2-3 weeks.
*Amebiasis or *Balantidiasis	1-4 day periods of diarrhea alternating with normal stools; often blood or mucous in stools; crampy abdominal pain; cysts in stool.	Often years.
*Schistosomiasis Mansoni	Fever; cough; urticaria; tender hepatomegaly and lymphadenopathy; splenomegaly; ascites; stool containing ova; South America, Africa, Middle East; repeated skin exposure to contaminated water.	Months.

CHRONIC OR RECURRENT DIARRHEA
(Continued)

DIAGNOSTIC CONSIDERATIONS	RELEVANT DATA BASE	COURSE
*Schistoso-miasis Japonicum	Enlarged tender liver; spenomegaly; repeated exposure to contaminated water; bloody stools; only in Far East; ova in stools.	Months.
*Strongyloi-diasis	Recurrent urticaria or blotchy red rash; cough, hemoptysis; larvae in stools.	Months.
*Trichuria-sis	Anemia; rectal prolapse; ova in stool.	Years.
*Fascio-lopsiasis	Ascites; mainly in China and India; ova in stools.	Years.
*Capillar-iasis	Voluminous watery diarrhea, malabsorption, muscle weakness and hyporeflexia; only in Phillipines; ova in stool.	Years.
*Tropical Sprue	Pale, malodorous, floating stools; postprandial abdominal discomfort, emotional lability; lassitude; sore tongue, emaciation; India, China, Far East, Central America.	Years.

*   Occur principally in persons who live, travel or have travelled in tropical or subtropical countries.

Reference: Harrison's Principles of Internal Medicine.   Seventh
             Edition.   Pages 215 - 217, 855, 1021.

HISTORY

Descriptors:

General descriptors: refer to inside cover.
   Is it progressive.
Location: exactly where food sticks.
Aggravating factors: solid or liquids.
Relieving factors: nitroglycerin ; regurgitation.
Past treatment or evaluation: past barium swallow; chest
   x-ray; gastroscopy.

Associated Symptoms:
Chest, neck or throat pain; regurgitation; neck swelling;
wheezing; hoarseness; cough; heart burn; weight loss;
anxiety; depression. Pediatric - drooling.

Medical History:
Raynaud's phenomenon; ulcers; hiatus hernia; neurological
disease; recent or recurrent pneumonia.

Environmental History:
History of swallowing chemicals; nasogastric intubation in
the past.

PHYSICAL EXAMINATION

Measure: weight.
Throat: check for signs of inflammation, swelling, asymetry;
   check gag reflex. (DO NOT use a tongue blade when examining
   the throat of a child with a sore throat and drooling).
Neck: check for any masses.

DIAGNOSTIC CONSIDERATIONS	HISTORY	PHYSICAL EXAM
OROPHARYNGEAL		
Muscle disease, neurological, or invasive disease	Discomfort in throat; occasional coughing due to aspiration on swallowing; cancers or neurological disease may be causative.	Structural abnormalities may rarely be noted in the throat or neck. Gag reflex may be abnormal.

DIAGNOSTIC CONSIDERATIONS	HISTORY	PHYSICAL EXAM
OROPHARYNGEAL		
Inflammation (pharyngitis, peritonsilar abscess, epiglottitis).	A severe sore throat may make swallowing painful. Pediatric - drooling.	Throat inflammation, asymetry, swelling or epiglottitis enlargement.
Unclear (Globus Hystericus)	"Lump in throat"; no difficulty swallowing.	Normal.
ESOPHAGEAL		
Propulsive abnormalities	Liquids and solids may cause regurgitation, "catching" in chest.	Usually normal.
Achalasia	Trouble swallowing liquids and solids; occasional pain relief from regurgitation.	Usually normal.
Diffuse spasm	Severe retrosternal pain often related to eating; relieved by nitroglycerin .	Usually normal.
Structural abnormalities	Often rapid progression of trouble swallowing - solids more often than liquids;may cause regurgitation at night and recurrent pulmonary infections.	Often leads to weight loss.

DIAGNOSTIC CONSIDERATIONS	HISTORY	PHYSICAL EXAM
Structural abnormalities (continued)		
Stricture	Heartburn may precede the trouble swallowing by years. Ingestion of corrosives may cause acute scarring of the esophagus; regurgitation may occur often.	Usually normal.
Tumor	Retrosternal chest pain; markedly progressive symptoms; eventual regurgitation of oral secretions.	Weight loss.
Scleroderma	Raynaud's phenomenon; heartburn common.	Variable.
Diverticula	Foul breath; regurgitation of food many hours after a meal; mild chest discomfort.	Normal.
Unclear (functional)	Trouble swallowing liquids but not solids. Poorly defined non-progressive symptoms not consistent with the causes listed above.	Normal.

Reference: Harrison's Principles of Internal Medicine. Seventh Edition. Pages 206 - 207.

HISTORY

Descriptors:

General descriptors: refer to inside cover.
Onset: relation to menses.
Character: color of discharge and amount.
Aggravating factors: sexual contact with persons having
  venereal disease; possible foreign body in vagina; preg-
  nancy.
Past treatment or evaluation: past evaluation; pelvic exam
  or pap test.

Associated Symptoms:

Fever or chills; abdominal pain; perineal pruritis; redness
or tenderness of vulva; foul odor of discharge; dysuria; skin
rash; joint pains; rectal pruritis (pediatric).

Medical History:

Gonorrhea; syphilis; vaginitis; diabetes.

Medications:

Oral contraceptives; antibiotics.

Environmental History:

Douching; sexual contact with persons having venereal disease;
possible foreign body in vagina.

PHYSICAL EXAMINATION

Abdomen: mass or tenderness.
Genital: Pelvic exam - cervical or adnexal tenderness; color
  and consistancy of discharge.
Special: pap test.

DIAGNOSTIC CONSIDERATIONS	HISTORY	PHYSICAL EXAM
Blood (See ABORTION or VAGINAL BLEEDING PROBLEMS)		
Candida (monilia)	More common in patients who are diabetic, pregnant, or taking oral contraceptives or antibiotics; often concurrent groin pruritis; white discharge minimal in amount.	White, curdy discharge on red base; overall vaginal mucosa often markedly inflamed. Small pustules may extend beyond the markedly inflamed area.

DIAGNOSTIC CONSIDERATIONS	HISTORY	PHYSICAL EXAM
Gonorrhea	Concurrent abdominal pain, fever, chills and joint pains are rarely noted. History of sexual contact with a person who has venereal disease.	Cervical or adnexal tenderness; green or yellow discharge may be seen issuing from cervical os.
Mixed bacteria	Often after history of excessive douching; occasionally an obstructing foreign body in the vagina; foul odor is usually present; minimal pruritis.	Foul smelling discharge. Vaginal mucosa often normal.
Trichomonas	Severe pruritis with profuse discharge. Odor often present.	Vaginal mucosa inflamed; discharge is frothy, gray, green or yellow.

Others:

Endometritis Cancer	Minimal discharge, at times bloody.	Abdominal and uterine masses or tenderness may be present.

Pediatric Considerations:

A clear discharge may occasionally be noted in normal girls. A foreign body in the vagina may result in a mixed bacterial infection with discharge; candida or pin worms may cause vaginal discharge and/or pruritis.

HISTORY

Descriptors:

General descriptors: refer to inside cover.
Onset: does patient describe a sensation of movement, rotation or spinning involving either the patient or the environment; how long have episodes been occuring; how long does an episode last.
Aggravating factors: position change; head turning; coughing; urination; standing suddenly.

Associated Symptoms:

Numbness in digits or around the mouth; anxiety or depression; double vision; loss of hearing or tinnitus; numbness; loss of strength or sensation; uncoordination; nausea or vomiting; melena; palpitations.

Medical History:

Anxiety or depression; hypertension; diabetes; cardiovascular disease; anemia; Meniere's disease; neurological disease; ear disease.

Medications:

Aspirin; alcohol; antihypertensives (particularly guanethedine (Ismelin); diuretics, diphenylhydantoin (Dilantin).

PHYSICAL EXAMINATION

Measure: blood pressure: standing and lying.
Ears: hearing; Rinne and Weber tests (Described under EAR PROBLEMS).
Eyes: nystagmus; visual acuity.
Neurological: cranial nerves; rapid rhythmic alternating movements; tandem gait; finger to nose tests; strength and sensation of extremities; deep tendon reflexes.
Special: Valsalva maneuver; hyperventilation for 3 minutes. Have seated patient suddenly lie flat; turn head rapidly; note if either of these motions may cause vertigo or nystagmus.

DIAGNOSTIC CONSIDERATIONS	HISTORY	PHYSICAL EXAM
(Actual loss of consciousness - See BLACKOUT)		

DIAGNOSTIC CONSIDERATIONS	HISTORY	PHYSICAL EXAM
<u>VERTIGO</u>	The patient perceives a sensation of movement, rotation or spinning involving either the patient or the environment.	
Central vertigo (Brain stem injury)	Acute onset of unilateral weakness, uncoordination, diplopia and numbness; usually not associated with nausea and vomiting.	Hearing often normal; neurological abnormalities noted, particularly vertical nystagmus.
Peripheral Vertigo		
Labyrinthitis	Acute attack of vertigo often with nausea and vomiting; usually lasts only a few days; occasionally recurrent.	Hearing normal; nystagmus during the attack.
Meniere's Disease	Often recurrent attacks of nausea, vomiting, tinnitis and vertigo with eventual decreased hearing.	Hearing decreased (neural deficit); horizontal nystagmus during attacks.
Positional	Acute vertigo usually present only on change of position or turning head quickly.	Rapid head positioning may cause nystagmus (often rotary nystagmus).
Acoustic Neuroma	Chronic progressive unilateral hearing deficit with tinnitis and occasional disequilibrium and vertigo.	Hearing loss (neural deficit) often accompanied by abnormalities of gait, cranial nerves 5, 7 and 10, and finger to nose tests on the same side.

DIAGNOSTIC CONSIDERATIONS	HISTORY	PHYSICAL EXAM
GIDDINESS	Lightheadedness; no sense of movement or rotation.	
Hyperventilation	Often symptoms of hyperventilation (tingling in fingers and around mouth) in the anxious or depressed patient.	Hyperventilation may reproduce symptoms; examination is otherwise normal.
Giddiness with multiple sensory deficits	Older patients who continually note dizziness when executing a sharp turn; patients are often diabetic.	Peripheral neuropathy and decreased vision due to cataracts are common.
Orthostatic giddiness	Patient may be on antihypertensive medications or have severe anemia; melena may be reported in the patient who has suffered gastrointestinal bleeding.	Orthostatic hypotension.
Giddiness during micturation, valsalva, coughing	The history suggests these as etiologic factors for giddiness.	These maneuvers may reproduce the symptoms.
Other		
(Less specific causes of dizziness)		
Drug intoxication (alcohol, diphenylhydantoin, aspirin, sedatives).	Tinnitus often noted with aspirin.	Nystagmus and disequilibrium may be present.

DIAGNOSTIC CONSIDERATIONS	HISTORY	PHYSICAL EXAM
Other		
Ocular abnormalities	Decreased or double vision may be noted.	Strabismus or extra-ocular movement ab-normalities may be present.
Chronic ear disease	Decreased hearing due to recurrent ear in-fections may be noted.	Decreased hearing (conductive type).

Reference: Harrison's Principles of Internal Medicine. Seventh
            Edition. Pages 94 - 96.

HISTORY

Descriptors:

General descriptors: refer to inside cover.
Note if it is constant or only after prolonged use of eyes.
Does the patient complain of double vision or being cross
eyed. Was the onset acute. Was there head or eye trauma.
Location: is the double vision noted with both eyes or one
eye only; which eye deviates; is it in all fields of gaze.
Aggravating factors: what direction of vision accentuates
diplopia.

Associated Symptoms:

Headache; eye pain; change in visual acuity; deviation of
eyes; protuberance of eyes; any trouble speaking; any unsteadiness on feet; any motor or sensory change elsewhere.

Medical History:

Thyroid disease; diabetes; high blood pressure; neurological disease; cerebrovascular disease.

Medications:

Any.

Family History:

Squint, crossed eyes, or wall eyes.

False Positive Considerations:

Blurred vision alone. (See EYE PROBLEMS).

PHYSICAL EXAMINATION

Measure: blood pressure.
Eyes: visual acuity; check extraocular movements; direction
of vision that accentuates diplopia; funduscopic exam.
Neurological: cranial nerves.
Special: have patient look at a distant point and alternately
cover and uncover each eye; watch for movement of the eye
being uncovered.

GENERAL CONSIDERATIONS

The person with blurred vision frequently claims double
vision (for blurred vision See EYE PROBLEMS). On the other
hand children may have obvious deviation of the eyes and not
complain of double vision. (See EYE PROBLEMS - amblyopia).

DIAGNOSTIC CONSIDERATIONS	HISTORY	PHYSICAL EXAM

Eye Muscle Dysfunction

Direct functional impairment (tumor; trauma; pressure of exophthalmic thyroid diseases).	May note exophthalmos, eye pain; double vision present in certain directions; history of trauma may be noted.	Exophthalmos often noted. Fixed ocular deviation or impairment of movement may be noted. Light reflexes and visual acuity often normal.
Strabismus (Eye muscle imbalance, crossed eye, wall-eye, squint)	Eyes turn in or out, sometimes worse when tired; may be family history; may be poor vision in one eye; diplopia rare except with intermittent cases, or acute causes (such as trauma).	Strabismus may be apparent on inspection or only during the cover-uncover test; poor vision in one eye (requires treatment at young age--see EYE PROBLEMS - amblyopia).

Peripheral Cranial Nerve Disease

(intra-cranial aneurysm; diabetes)	Headache and pain behind the eye may be noted.	One or both eye movements will be limited in at least one direction. In diabetes the pupil response may be normal.
Trauma	See Direct functional impairment above.	

Brain Stem Disease

	Trouble walking or speaking; vertigo; motor dysfunctions may be present.	Multiple cranial nerve abnormalities are usually noted. Nystagmus is common.

DIAGNOSTIC CONSIDERATIONS	HISTORY	PHYSICAL EXAM

Other:

| Myasthenia Gravis | Muscle weakness, trouble talking, and double vision often more troublesome as the day progresses. | Ptosis often present. Patient has difficulty in carrying out repetitive movement. |

Causes of blurred vision may occasionally make the patient claim double vision. (See EYE PROBLEMS).

Reference: Harrison's Principles of Internal Medicine. Seventh Edition. Pages 104 - 106.

HISTORY

Descriptors:

General descriptors: refer to inside cover.
Location: unilateral or bilateral ear problems.
Past treatment or evaluation: previous hearing test or other
   evaluation.

Associated Symptoms:

Headache; nausea and vomiting; fever or chills; ear pain;
hearing loss; ear discharge; ringing or buzzing in ears;
runny nose; sore throat; sensation of movement or rotation;
loss of equilibrium.

Medical History:

High blood pressure; neurological disease; anxiety; depression;
Meniere's disease; ear infections; severe head trauma; mumps.

Medications:

Aspirin; streptomycin; diuretics; quinine.

Family History:

Hearing trouble.

Environmental History:

Ear trouble noted after swimming or bathing; noisy environment; possibility of a foreign body in the ear.

PHYSICAL EXAMINATION

Pediatric:

age 0-3 months - note if there is a response to noise.
age 3-5 months - note if the child turns to sound.
age 6-10 months - note if the child responds to name.
age 10-15 months - note if the child imitates simple words.

Ears: check hearing with watch tick. Check external canal and
   tympanic membrane; note if tympanic membranes move from the
   pressure of the pneumatic otoscope.
Neurological: check sensation of face; note if patient's smile
   is symmetrical; perform finger to nose test.
Special: place a vibrating tuning fork in the middle of the
   forehead, ask the patient if the sound is best heard on one
   side or the other (Weber test).
      Place a vibrating tuning fork over the mastoid process, note
   if the patient hears the tuning fork longer when placed next
   to his ear than when on the mastoid process (Rinne test).

DIAGNOSTIC CONSIDERATIONS	HISTORY	PHYSICAL EXAM
DECREASED HEARING		
CHRONIC		
Conductive Hearing Loss	Loss of hearing for all frequencies.	In unilateral disease Rinne test shows air conduction less than bone conduction. The Weber test lateralizes to the involved ear.
Otosclerosis	Old Age.	Ear exam otherwise normal.
Ear Wax or Foreign Body		Ear exam reveals wax or foreign body; hearing returns when they are removed.
Chronic otitis externa, serous otitis	Decreased hearing in the young child; a foul ear discharge may be noted.	Decreased mobility of the tympanic membrane; discharge, tympanic membrane perforation and cholesteatoma may be present.
Nerve Deficit Type hearing loss	High frequency hearing loss is often noted. Thus, the patient may note difficulty when speaking on the telephone.	In unilateral disease both air and bone conduction are decreased. The Weber test lateralizes to the uninvolved ear.
Presbycusis	Old Age.	Ear exam otherwise normal.
Loss Secondary to chronic noise, severe head trauma or mumps	A history of these factors is obtained.	Usually normal. If severe head trauma, ear discharge or temporal bone tenderness may be present.

DIAGNOSTIC CONSIDERATIONS	HISTORY	PHYSICAL EXAM

DECREASED HEARING

CHRONIC (continued)

Nerve Deficit Type hearing loss

Secondary to acoustic neuroma	Decreased hearing; Tinnitus may be noted.	Decreased hearing; abnormal sensation of face, finger to nose test or movement of facial musculature on the involved side.
Secondary to ototoxic medications	History of prolonged treatment with ethacrynic acid, furosemide, streptomycin, Kanamycin or quinine. Tinnitus is common.	Exam is otherwise normal.
Congenital	Deafness (usually bilateral) since birth. A family history of deafness may be present; delayed speech is common.	Usually normal though other defects may be present.

DECREASED HEARING

ACUTE

Associated with ear pain or discharge, See below.

Associated with the sensation of movement or rotation, See DIZZINESS - VERTIGO.

Secondary to trauma, See Nerve Deficit Hearing Loss above.

DIAGNOSTIC CONSIDERATIONS	HISTORY	PHYSICAL EXAM

EAR PAIN or DISCHARGE

Otitis Media	Ear pain; decreased hearing; often follows an upper respiratory infection.	Fever; decreased mobility of tympanic membrane; tympanic membrane is often inflammed and may be bulging; decreased air conductive hearing.
Otitis Externa	Ear pain; discharge is usually present; may follow swimming; decreased hearing may be noted.	Fever; extremely tender, inflammed and exudative ear canal; normal tympanic membrane.
Acute Mastoiditis	Usually follows acute otitis media.	Exquisite tenderness or fluctuance over the mastoid process.
Chronic Otitis Externa or Media	Persistant foul smelling ear discharge with decreased hearing; little ear pain is noted.	Discharge is common; abnormal tympanic membrane or external canal; tympanic membrane does not respond to pneumo-otoscopic pressure.

TINNITUS
(Ringing or buzzing in ears)

Associated with sensation of movement or rotation, See DIZZINESS - VERTIGO.

Associated with any of the causes of decreased hearing, ear pain or discharge, See above.

Secondary to high dose aspirin	High dose aspirin ingestion.	Normal.
Unclear	A nervous person may complain of Tinnitus. No hearing loss is noted.	Normal.

Reference: Harrison's Principles of Internal Medicine. Seventh Edition. Pages 105-108.

HISTORY

Descriptors:

General descriptors: refer to inside cover.
How does the patient judge his eating as excessive (i.e., com-
pared to whom). Exactly how much of what type of food is eaten
each day. Are all meals of equivalent size; how many meals per
day; eating between meals.

Associated Symptoms:
Anxiety; depression; eating to relieve emotional stress; change
in weight; excessive urination or excessive thirst; heat intolerance; weakness.

Medical History:
Diabetes; thyroid disease; emotional disease; obesity.

PHYSICAL EXAMINATION

Measure: weight; height.
Eyes: does the sclera above the cornea become apparent when
eyes follow an object inferiorly; exophthalmos.
Neck: enlarged or nodular thyroid.

GENERAL CONSIDERATIONS

Excessive eating is a common complaint of the obese; it also
occurs in people with hyperthyroidism or uncontrolled diabetes
(See THYROID TROUBLE or DIABETES). The range of normal daily
caloric intake for a moderately active adult is 2200-2800
calories for men and 1800-2100 calories for women who are not
pregnant or lactating.

HISTORY

Descriptors:

General descriptors: refer to inside cover.
How much does the patient drink; what is the usual volume
of urine output per day; amount of each voiding; how frequently is the patient awakened at night by the desire to
drink or urinate.
Aggravating factors: alcohol or coffee drinking; diuretic
  therapy.

Associated Symptoms:

Anxiety/depression; headaches; orthopnea; dysuria; fever;
chills; dribbling or change in force of urine stream; nocturia;
frequency; excessive eating; swelling of extremities.

Medical History:

Diabetes; anxiety/depressive illness; neurological disease;
intracranial surgery or skull fractures; kidney disease;
urinary tract infections; prostate disease; cardiovascular
disease; liver disease.

Medications:

Diuretics; insulin or oral hypoglycemic agents.

Family History:

Diabetes.

False Positive Considerations:

Toddlers learning to control urination may have to pass urine
frequently and urgently.

PHYSICAL EXAMINATION

Measure: weight; blood pressure - standing and lying; pulse;
  temperature.
Eyes: fundi- hemorrhages, exudate, papilledema, or microaneurysms.
Chest: rales.
Heart: murmurs, gallops or enlargement.
Extremities: pitting edema.

GENERAL CONSIDERATIONS

Generally, the body's fluid equilibrium is maintained by
a balance between fluid intake and urinary output. Therefore, in the setting of polydipsia one must consider causes
of polyuria - and vice versa.

Urine output covers a wide range of normal. The average
daily adult urine output is 1.5 liters and the average child
over 15 kilograms puts out about 30-50 ccs per kilogram per
day. A urinary output of more than 5 liters per day should
always be regarded as abnormal.

Frequency of urination without increase in actual amount
of urine is a common complaint of persons with urinary tract
infections or partial obstruction of urinary outflow as in
benign prostatic hypertrophy (see URINE TROUBLES).

Normal adults usually do not awaken from sleep in order to
void (nocturia) unless they have taken coffee, alcohol or
excessive amounts of fluid before going to bed. Children
often urinate at night until bladder control is adequate
(see BEDWETTING).

DIAGNOSTIC CONSIDERATIONS	HISTORY	PHYSICAL EXAM
Polydipsia-Polyuria		
Uncontrolled diabetes mellitus	May have weight loss, family history of diabetes; excessive eating; nocturia.	Weight loss, decreased skin turgor may be present; microaneurysus in retinal vessels.
Diabetes insipidus	Patient has insatiable thirst day and night with urine output often exceeding 5 liters a day; may follow head trauma, neurological disease, or intracranial surgery.	Usually normal; may have papilledema or decreased skin turgor and orthostatic hypotension.

DIAGNOSTIC CONSIDERATIONS	HISTORY	PHYSICAL EXAM
Polydipsia-Polyuria		
Diuretic therapy	Taking a diuretic for heart disease or hypertension; nocturia.	Depends on underlying disease for which diuretics have been prescribed.
Chronic Renal Disease	A history of chronic renal disease; nocturia; weakness and orthostatic faintness may be noted if the patient is unable to drink enough fluid.	Physical exam is often normal; hypertension may be present.
"Psychogenic"	The anxious or depressed patient may complain of polydipsia and polyuria but is usually able to sleep through the night without drinking or urinating.	Normal.
Nocturia (also see above)		
Secondary to partial urethral obstruction (usually benign prostatic hypertrophy).	Older male. Difficulty initiating voiding; frequency; dribbling; decreased force of urinary stream.	Prostate often enlarged but may be normal size.

DIAGNOSTIC CONSIDERATIONS	HISTORY	PHYSICAL EXAM

Nocturia

Secondary to edematous states (heart failure, severe liver or renal disease)	Orthopnea; ankle swelling.	Pitting edema is present.

Reference: Harrison's Principles of Internal Medicine. Seventh Edition. Pages 243 - 244.

HISTORY

Descriptors:

General descriptors: refer to inside cover.
Aggravating factors: eye trauma or foreign body; contact lenses.
Past treatment or evaluation: has tonometry or eye examination been performed recently.

Associated Symptoms:
Visual loss or blurring; eye pain; eye redness or discharge; photophobia; double vision; tearing or dryness; lid irritation or swelling; halos about lights; headache.

Medical History:
Diabetes; hypertension; atherosclerosis; connective tissue disease; neurological disease; previous eye disease; migraine headaches; allergies (specify).

Medications:
Eye drops or ointment; adrenal steroids; thioridazine (Mellaril); chloroquine; Ethambutol (Myambutol); contact lenses.

Family History:
Glaucoma; other eye disease; diabetes.

Environmental History:
Exposure to toxins (wood alcohol, smog, etc.); dust; metal work (welding).

PHYSICAL EXAMINATION

Measure: blood pressure.
Eyes: check visual acuity pupil equality and reaction to light; extraocular movement; lids and conjunctiva noting pattern of inflammation; check cornea for abrasions and fundus for hemorrhages, exudates, cup to disc ratio and papilledema.
Special: if visual acuity is abnormal, have the patient look at the chart through a pinhole and note if vision is improved.
If the patient complains of a foreign body and none is apparent, examine the everted lids; topically anesthetize the eye and examine using fluorescein.

PHYSICAL EXAMINATION
(Continued)

Special, preventative screening:
Pediatric only: have child look at a distant point and
    alternately cover and uncover each eye; watch for movement
    of the eye being uncovered. If the infant is too young
    to check vision, note the symmetry of a light reflection
    on the cornea.
        Amblyopia must be detected before the child is 6-8 years
    of age or visual loss is irreversible. The younger the
    patient, the easier to treat.

Adult only: perform tonometry unless the eye is inflamed or
    injured.
        Glaucoma (open angle) is common over the age of 40. Mea-
    surement of tonometry and the cup to disc ratio consti-
    tutes effective screening for this cause of blindness. By
    the time visual abnormalities are noted by the patient,
    severe irreversible damage has already occured (see Blurred
    Vision below).

GENERAL CONSIDERATIONS

Cautions:
    Do not prescribe topical anesthetics for home use; eye
damage can result.
    Do not do tonometry on infected or injured eyes.
    Allow no pressure upon any eye which might be perforated.
Protect the eye with a dressing or shield braced on the brow
and cheek.
    Never try to dislodge a deeply imbedded foreign body.
    Irrigate a chemical injury before doing anything else.
Alkalis require 30 minutes of irrigation.
    Definitive treatment for sudden blindness, acute angle
closure glaucoma, eye perforation and corneal ulcer must be
begun as soon as possible or permanent severe eye damage will
result.

DIAGNOSTIC CONSIDERATIONS	HISTORY	PHYSICAL EXAM
EMERGENCIES		
Sudden Blindness	Acute, painless visual loss; sometimes as if veil descended.	Unreactive or sluggish pupil; retinal pallor (arterial occlusion), hemorrhage or detachment.
Acute Glaucoma (angle closure)	Painful red eye often with headache, nausea and vomiting. May be precipitated by mydriatics, darkness, stress. Blurred vision; halo around lights.	Mid-dilated unreactive pupil. Inflamed eye; steamy cornea. Increased tonometric pressure and shallow anterior chamber. (Note: tonometry may be normal between attacks).
Corneal Ulcer (bacterial)	Sore red eye; blurred vision; photophobia; often history of scratch or foreign body.	Whitish or yellowish ulcer on cornea; often pus settling in anterior chamber. Severe iritis.
Chemical Injury	Chemical struck eyes.	WASH OUT INSTANTLY-- damage can occur in seconds, and continues while chemical is in eye. Ask questions later; examine later.
Penetrating Injury	Often trauma known; sometimes patient only recalls a speck in the eye; history of hammering or grinding or using power tools. Usually but not always eye pain.	The foreign body is usually obvious but entry site can be small or partially self-sealing.

DIAGNOSTIC CONSIDERATIONS	HISTORY	PHYSICAL EXAM
BLURRED VISION (see also EMERGENCIES)		
(when the eye is not inflamed)		
Refractive error (patients less than 45 years of age).	Poor vision, often worse in one eye; must sit close to movie screen, blackboard etc.	Decreased visual acuity; improved looking through pinhole.
Amblyopia (Pediatric)	Poor vision in one eye; eyes may turn in or out.	Decreased visual acuity in one eye, not improved by looking through pinhole. Strabismus may be apparent on inspection or only during the cover-uncover test.
Cataracts	Usually elderly patients. Painless gradual loss of vision. May be accelerated in those taking chronic adrenal steroids or having previous eye disease.	Cataract in lens.
Presbyopia (patients over 45 years of age)	Difficulty reading; the patient must hold objects far away in order to see them clearly.	Good visual acuity for distant objects.
Chronic (open angle Glaucoma)	Usually asymptomatic until blurred vision or loss of peripheral vision indicate irreversible eye damage.	Increased tonometric pressure. Cup to disc ratio more than 0.5.

DIAGNOSTIC CONSIDERATIONS	HISTORY	PHYSICAL EXAM
BLURRED VISION (continued) (when the eye is not inflamed)		
Toxic Drugs	Eyedrops.	Pupil may be very large or small and unreactive; accomodation is often abnormal.
	Retino-toxic drugs (chloroquine, thioridazine, ethambutol).	Decreased visual acuity; funduscopic examination may show pigment changes.
Retino-vascular	Diabetes; hypertension; atherosclerosis.	Retinal degeneration, hemorrhages or exudates are usually present; decreased visual acuity; papilledema may be present.

INFLAMED (RED) EYE (see also EMERGENCIES)

Simple conjunctivitis ("allergic", bacterial or viral).	Eyelid feels as though sand were present; eyes burn and tear; mild blurred vision and photophobia. May occasionally be caused by allergies, upper respiratory infections or connective tissue diseases.	Injection inside lids and peripherally on eyeball. Allergies may cause conjunctival edema.

DIAGNOSTIC CONSIDERATIONS	HISTORY	PHYSICAL EXAM
INFLAMED (RED) EYE (Continued)		
Acute Iritis	Photophobia; the eye is often very sore and aching; vision is usually blurred.	Circumcorneal injection or flush; pupil may be small and weakly reactive; the anterior chamber may be hazy. Foreign bodies may rarely be present.
Herpes simplex kerato-conjuncti-vitis	Photophobia; the eye may be sore or 'feel like sand is present'.	Fluorescein staining reveals corneal lesions; also conjunctivitis and occasionally iritis.

Acute angle closure glaucoma: see EMERGENCIES.

FOREIGN BODY/TRAUMA   (see also Emergencies above)

Conjunctival foreign body	The eye feels as though "something is in it." History of speck flying into the eye.	Foreign body on white of eye or under everted lids.
Corneal abrasion or foreign body	Painful and photophobic eye. History of speck flying into the eye or wearing contact lenses.	Fluorescein staining reveals corneal abrasion or foreign body.
Blunt Injury	Struck in eye. Vision may be blurred or double.	Changes consistent with iritis may be present. Rarely blood may be present in the anterior chamber. Rarely eye movement may be limited and the orbital bones fractured.

DIAGNOSTIC CONSIDERATIONS	HISTORY	PHYSICAL EXAM
LID PROBLEMS		
Sty	Painful pustule on lid.	Lid pustule.
Allergies	Red, itchy lids; tearing.	Red or swollen lids without discharge or tenderness.
Blepharitis	Chronic red, dry, itchy irritated lids, especially at lash margins.	Reddened, thickened lid margins with crusting of material in lashes.
Chronic Tearing (Epiphora)	Tears run continuously. May note 'allergies'.	Eye inspection may demonstrate lid laxity (ectropion) or swollen (plugged) lacrimal sac.
Dacryocystitis	Swollen tender skin near medial canthus.	Swollen red tissue over lacrimal sac; purulent discharge may be present.
OTHER EYE SYMPTOMS		
Double Vision	See DOUBLE VISION	
Squint / Strabismus	See Amblyopia above.	
Stroke; Tumor; Intracranial disease	Painless visual deficit (often without patient awareness) or transient loss of vision ; occasionally referred pain to the eye or headache.	Abnormal visual fields, pupillary or eye movements are often present. Nystagmus may occur.
Tic douloureux	Jabs of pain, often about eye; patient may note trigger areas that cause pain.	Usually normal.

DIAGNOSTIC CONSIDERATIONS	HISTORY	PHYSICAL EXAM

OTHER EYE SYMPTOMS (Continued)

DIAGNOSTIC CONSIDERATIONS	HISTORY	PHYSICAL EXAM
Classic Migraine Headache	The patient sees transient "spots" or flashing lights followed by a unilateral headache.	Normal.
Proptosis-secondary to orbital tumor	Prominent eye; decrease visual acuity; double vision.	Unilateral exophthalmos; decrease visual acuity; funduscopic examination often reveals optic atrophy of papilledema.

HISTORY

Descriptors:

General descriptors: refer to inside cover.
Location: precisely where is the pain located.
Aggravating factors: does touching any area trigger attacks of pain.
Relieving factors: is pain relieved by standing.

Associated Symptoms:
Headaches; recent facial trauma; anxiety; depression; fever; ear ache; eye pain; visual change; nasal discharge; tooth ache.

Medical History:
Diabetes; migraine headaches; any neurological disease; recurrent ear infection; rheumatoid arthritis; glaucoma; sinus disease; dental infections.

Medications:
Diphenylhydantoin (Dilantin); ergot derivatives (Cafergot); codeine; aspirin; other treatment for pain.

Family History:
Family history of headaches.

PHYSICAL EXAMINATION

Measure: temperature.
Head: check for sinus tenderness; search for areas of face where touching causes pain; check sensation over face to pinprick and vibration; look for a vesicular skin eruption.
Ears: check for tympanic membrane discoloration or perforation.
Eyes: check the pupillary response to light and accomodation; injection of conjunctivae.
Throat: dental hygiene; percuss the teeth on side of pain.

DIAGNOSTIC CONSIDERATIONS	HISTORY	PHYSICAL EXAM
Acute		
Acute Sinusitis	Nasal congestion and discharge; pain improves with standing.	Fever; sinus tenderness; erythema and edema may overlie the painful area; purulent nasal discharge.

DIAGNOSTIC CONSIDERATIONS	HISTORY	PHYSICAL EXAM
Acute		
Glaucoma (acute angle closure)	Painful red eye often with headache, nausea and vomiting. May be precipitated by mydriatics, darkness, or stress. Blurred vision; halo around lights.	Mid dilated unreactive pupil. Inflamed eye; steamy cornea; shallow anterior chamber.
Dental Abscess	Toothache	Poor dental hygiene; tooth is tender to direct percussion.
Chronic/recurrent		
Tic Douloureux	Brief "jabs" of unilateral severe pain. Precipitated by hot, cold, or pressure over "trigger" area.	Pressure over certain areas of the face may induce an attack of pain.
Temporo mandibular joint pain	Pain on chewing. History of rheumatoid arthritis.	Crepitation and tenderness may be noted over the temporo-mandibular joint.
Herpes Zoster	Continuous unilateral facial pain preceding, following or during a unilateral vesicular skin eruption.	Unilateral vesicular eruption which ends in the midline and is confined to one or more dermatomes.
Chronic or acute otitis media.	Ear ache and decreased hearing may be noted.	Perforated, inflamed or thickened tympanic membrane.
Migraine Headache.	See HEADACHE.	

HISTORY

Descriptors:

General descriptors: refer to inside cover.
Pattern of temperature elevation; what was the temperature.

Aggravating factors: Pediatric - immunization within 3 days
of this visit.

Associated Symptoms:
Shaking chills; change in weight; night sweats; headache;
stiff neck; ear pain or ear pulling; sore throat; chest
pain; cough; sputum production; trouble breathing; abdominal
pain; urinary frequency; dysuria or crying on urination
(pediatric); dark urine; bone or joint pain; skin rash
or pustules.

Medical History:
Valvular heart disease; diabetes; tuberculosis; mononucleosis; positive tuberculin test.

Medications:
Steroids; any other.

Environmental History:
Foreign travel in last 6 months; contact with patients with
tuberculous pneumonia; recent contact with persons with
streptococcal pharyngitis, upper respiratory illness, or
the gastrointestinal "flu" syndrome.
Tick bite within the last 2 weeks.
Pediatric: was the child in excessively warm clothing
when the temperature was obtained.

PHYSICAL EXAMINATION

Measure: rectal temperature, pulse, weight, blood pressure.

Perform a complete physical examination if there are no
localizing symptoms. Note Carefully:

Head: sinus tenderness; Pediatric - bulging fontanel.
Ears: tympanic membrane - inflammation, bulging, loss of
landmarks or lack of movement to pneumatic otoscope.
Throat: pharyngeal inflammation; Pediatric - small white
specks on the oral mucosa.
Neck: stiffness.
Chest: rales or localized rhonchi and wheezes.
Heart: murmurs.

PHYSICAL EXAMINATION

Abdomen: tenderness; flanks - punch tenderness.
Extremities: swelling, redness or tenderness of legs.
Skin: petechiae; pustules or abscesses; any rash.
Nodes: lymphadenopathy.

GENERAL CONSIDERATIONS (Adult)

Fever accompanies many illnesses and may be the first manifestation of diseases which usually present in other ways.

Listed below are the common generally acute, benign causes
of fever followed by some of the serious (often fatal if
not treated) diseases which may present with fever.

DIAGNOSTIC CONSIDERATIONS (ADULT)	HISTORY	PHYSICAL EXAM
Upper respiratory illness/ pharyngitis	Sore throat; runny nose; cough with non-purulent sputum; contact with others with the same problem.	Mild fever; often mild throat inflammation noted.
Mononucleosis	Persistent sore throat; lethargy. No prior history of mononucleosis.	Severely inflamed pharynx; posterior cervical or generalized adenopathy; splenomegaly occasionally.
"Flu" syndrome	Muscle aches and pains; nausea; vomiting and diarrhea; loss of appetite; malaise; history of others with the same problem.	Mild fever; minimal abdominal tenderness.
Urinary tract infection	Frequency; dysuria; flank ache; hematuria may be noted. Urinary tract infections are often asymptomatic in the child.	Punch tenderness of flank may be present.

DIAGNOSTIC
CONSIDERATIONS (ADULT)   HISTORY   PHYSICAL EXAM

Drug fever   Any drug reaction may   Occasionally skin rash.
                      cause fever.

Serious Diseases Which   Usual Presenting Complaints
May Present With Fever   or Findings

Pneumonia   Cough; green or yellow sputum; chest
                              pain; localized abnormal findings on
                              lung exam.

Meningitis   Headache; stiff neck.

Intra-abdominal   Abdominal pain, tenderness or mass.
abscess   Recent abdominal surgery.

Neoplasm   Fatigue; weight loss; lymphadeno-
                              pathy; masses often present.

Osteomyelitis   Bone pain, tenderness, and swelling;
                              muscle spasm.

Septic Arthritis   Usually monoarticular joint swelling.

Tuberculosis   Cough; weight loss; night sweats; re-
                              cent contact with active tuberculosis
                              or a past history of positive tuber-
                              culin test.

Connective Tissue   Joint pains; headaches; skin rash;
Disease   pleuritic chest pain.

Bacterial   History of valvular heart disease,
Endocarditis   heart murmurs, petechiae and spleno-
                              megaly; dyspnea; weakness.

Thrombophlebitis   Leg pain, redness, swelling or
                              tenderness.

Rocky Mountain   Recent tick bite; purpuric skin le-
spotted fever   sions; headache.

Tropical infections   Recent travel or residence in a
(Malaria, Leishmaniasis,   tropical area; splenomegaly may be
 Chagas disease and   present.
 others)

GENERAL CONSIDERATIONS (Pediatric)

Children react with a dramatic febrile response to seemingly minor infections. Common causes of fever in children
are acute otitis media (ear ache, ear pulling), upper respiratory infections/ pharyngitis (cough, sore inflamed throat),
"flu" syndromes (nausea, vomiting and diarrhea) and the
response to immunization.

Less common causes of fever include any of the diagnostic
considerations of adults listed above.

Other causes of fever in children are:

Roseola: Three days of high fever in otherwise "well"
 child. Pink rash appears on 4th day and fever subsides.
Measles: Cough; fever; conjunctivitis and small whitish
 specks in the mouth. Three days later onset of raised
 rash which spreads over the entire body.
Rheumatic fever and juvenile rheumatoid arthritis: fever
 and joint pains are often noted.
Skin infections and scarlet fever: skin rash, pustules or
 abscesses.
Excessively warm clothing on a youngster may cause elevated
 temperature which returns to normal shortly after the
 clothes are removed.

Reference: Harrison's Principles of Internal Medicine. Seventh
 Edition. Pages 54 - 63.

HISTORY

Descriptors:

General descriptors: refer to inside cover.
Location: generalized or localized.
Character: aching or burning pain.
Aggravating factors: is the pain most noticeable during walk-
ing, standing or shoe wearing; was there foot or ankle trauma.
Past treatment or evaluation: past x-ray of foot or ankle;
past orthopedic evaluation.

Associated Symptoms:
Joint pains; numbness of foot.

Medical History:
Gout; alcoholism; pernicious anemia; diabetes; rheumatoid
arthritis.

Medications:
Colchicine; allopurinol (Zyloprim); probenecid (Benemid);
INH (Isoniazid).

PHYSICAL EXAMINATION

Extremities: Foot and ankle - tenderness; swelling; discoloration; deformity; change in range of motion; pain on
movement or weight bearing; calluses under metatarsal heads.
Squeeze forefoot to elicit pain if complaint involves
metatarsal area.
Have patient stand and observe the forefoot for splaying
on weight bearing.
Neurological: check sensation to pinprick or vibration over
toes.

Diagnostic considerations based on the location of foot or ankle discomfort.

Usual Location	Common Disease	Findings
Anterior foot	Foot strain	Aching following a change in occupation, shoes or activity; fore-foot may splay on weight bearing; if chronic, calluses are eventually noted under the meta-tarsal heads.

Usual Location	Common Disease	Findings
Anterior foot	Rheumatoid arthritis	Other chronic joint pains and deformity; marked prominence of the metatarsal heads and deformity of the forefoot is usually present.
Ankle	Traumatic Injury (sprain)	Usually a history of inversion injury; tenderness and swelling noted over the anterior talofibular ligament.
	Traumatic Injury (fracture)	Deformity; crepitus; localized tenderness, swelling, bruising, or abnormal mobility of a bone or joint.
Heel (adult)	Fasciitis	Aching or sharp pain often following stress. Deep tenderness noted over the ball of the heel.
	Achilles tendinitis or bursitis	Shoes may be noted to rub against the tender area; tenderness and swelling is noted over the lower achilles tendon.
Heel and midfoot (pediatric)	Osteochondritis	Ages 4-14. May follow injury. Tenderness noted by pressing over the posterior portion of the heel bone or the navicular bone.
Localized pain between 3rd and 4th metatarsals	(Probable neuroma)	Burning pain increased by squeezing of the forefoot.

FOOT - ANKLE PAIN
(Continued)

Usual Location	Common Disease	Findings
Great toe pain	Degenerative arthritis, stiff toe or bunion	Chronic pain with each step. Tender bunion and/or pain on extension of the great toe.
	Gout	Male patients over 40. Acute, often recurrent pain at the base of the great toe usually accompanied by pain in other joints. A red swollen tender base of the great toe is present.
Variable location, often entire sole.	Neuropathy	Burning pins and needles type pain. Common in diabetic and alcoholic patients. Decreased sensation in the foot is often present.

HISTORY

Descriptors:

General descriptors: refer to inside cover.
Onset: when was the frostbite noted.
Aggravating factors: was the exposed area wet - if yes, for
  how long; how many prior doses of tetanus toxoid has the
  patient received.

Associated Symptoms:
Is the exposed area numb, blue, white, or painful.

PHYSICAL EXAMINATION

Note the extent of involved area; check sensation in involved area.

GENERAL CONSIDERATIONS

Cold injury is intensified if the exposed area is also wet.
Initially one might note that areas exposed to cold are
blue. In severe, irreversible injury the involved area is
white and lacks sensitivity to pinprick. Any area that has
suffered true frostbite should be treated as a potentially
contaminated wound.

Reference: Harrison's Principles of Internal Medicine. Seventh
            Edition. Pages 53 - 54.

HISTORY

Descriptors:

General descriptors: refer to inside cover.
Aggravating factors: is problem worse in darkness or when
    trying to rise from a seated position.

Associated Symptoms:

Headache; tinnitis; any weakness or changes in sensation;
tremor; joint, back,neck or leg pain.

Medical History:

Alcoholism; diabetes; any neurological disease; chronic anemia;
syphillis; cerebrovascular disease; cerebral palsey; arthritis
or joint disease.

Medications:

Barbiturates; tranquilizers; anticonvulsants (Dilantin).

Family History:

Abnormal gait or coordination; hip disease (pediatric).

False Positive:

Orthostatic dizziness causing unsteadiness.

PHYSICAL EXAMINATION

Measure: blood pressure lying and standing.
Extremities: muscle strength; note manner of walking.
    Pediatric--note hip range of motion and measure leg length.
Neurological: deep tendon reflexes; vibratory sensation; heel
    to toe walking; finger-to-nose test; Romberg test.
Special (pediatric): standing on one foot; drawing figures.

DIAGNOSTIC CONSIDERATIONS	HISTORY	PHYSICAL EXAM
MUSCLE OR MOTOR SYSTEM DISEASE		
Weakness	Usually a chronic problem; family history of muscle weakness may be present; localized weakness may be secondary to nerve root compression in the neck or back causing leg, neck or back pain.	Muscle weakness noted; in legs there may be a waddle or flinging movement of the weak limb; difficulty rising from the seated position.
Spasticity	In adults often following a cerebrovascular accident or compression of the spinal cord in the neck or upper back; children frequently are mentally retarded (cerebral palsy); incontinence of stool or urine.	In the legs the spastic limb is swung around by hip action; Babinski reflex, hyperactive reflexes and distal weakness are present.
Minimal cerebral dysfunction (pediatric only)	"Clumsy child" with normal intelligence.	Fine motor coordination is often abnormal (standing on one foot, threading a needle, drawing); neurological examination is grossly normal.
CEREBELLAR, SENSORY OR BASAL GANGLIA DISEASE		
Sensory ataxia	Usually worse in the dark; may follow syphillis or pernicious anemia, but is most common in diabetes.	Decreased vibratory sense, position sense and ankle jerks in the legs; Romberg test is abnormal; gait is "stamping".

DIAGNOSTIC CONSIDERATIONS	HISTORY	PHYSICAL EXAM

CEREBELLAR, SENSORY OR BASAL GANGLIA DISEASE
(Continued)

Cerebellar ataxia	Tremor often noted; most often seen in alcoholics, but may be familial or a result of a brain tumor or cerebrovascular accident (headache, tinnitis, other defects are usually noted).	The Romberg test is normal but one or more of the following abnormalities is usually present: --Poor performance on rapidly rhythmic alternating movements, finger-to-nose testing or tandem walk. --Nystagmus. --Unsteady, wide-based gait.
Parkinsonian gait	Gradually progressive with resting tremor and difficulty initiating movement.	Shuffling gait; resting tremor which decreases with intention; cogwheel rigidity of arms; flexed posture; turns with a fixed body position; poor balance.
Intoxicated stagger	Excessive intake of alcohol, barbiturates or rarely tranquilizers; rarely anticonvulsants.	Generalized uncoordination and unsteadiness with little attempt to correct gait; memory is often poor.

ORTHOPEDIC DISEASE

Adult	Joint or limb pain.	See JOINT - EXTREMITY PAIN.
Pediatric, age 1-3 (usually congenital dislocated hips)	Limp without complaints of limb discomfort; usually a female child with a family history of hip disease.	Shortened leg with slight external rotation; hip range of motion is often decreased.

DIAGNOSTIC CONSIDERATION	HISTORY	PHYSICAL EXAM
ORTHOPEDIC DISEASE (Continued)		
Pediatric, age 5-16 (usually Perthe's disease or slipped femoral epiphysis)	Hip or knee pain may be noted; limp.	Decreased hip range of motion.
OTHER		
Hysterical gait	The patient is often relatively unconcerned by problem and seldom hurts himself despite claiming to fall frequently.	Inconsistent "abnormalities", exaggerated when being observed; staggering gait but does not fall.

Reference: Harrison's Principles of Internal Medicine. Seventh Edition. Pages 96-100.

HISTORY

Descriptors:

General descriptors: refer to inside cover.
Onset: acute or chronic.
Aggravating factors: does the patient rub, pull or scratch
    involved area; recent childbirth.

Associated Symptoms:
    Itching of involved area; axillary or pubic hair loss.
    If hair excess in female: menstrual irregularity, acne,
        voice change.

Medical History:
    Thyroid or adrenal disease; lupus erythematosis; psoriasis
    or other chronic skin diseases.

Medications:
    Adrenal steroids; anticoagulants; cancer chemotherapeutic
    agents.

Family History:
    Similar problem.

PHYSICAL EXAMINATION

Skin: any rashes; note carefully the character of the skin
    underlying any localized hair change; note if the hair is
    depigmented or thin; are there broken hair shafts.

DIAGNOSTIC CONSIDERATIONS	HISTORY	PHYSICAL EXAM
SPOTS OF SCALP HAIR LOSS:		
Fungus (Tinea)	Usually children; a-symptomatic localized loss of hair.	Bald spots with broken hairs.
Alopecia areate	Asymptomatic localized loss of hair.	Perfectly smooth areas without hair; hair may become depigmented.

DIAGNOSTIC CONSIDERATIONS	HISTORY	PHYSICAL EXAM
SPOTS OF SCALP HAIR LOSS: (Continued)		
Secondary to skin disease (psoriasis, seborrheic dermatitis, lupus erythematosis, infection)	History of other skin lesions or pruritus often noted.	Underlying skin lesions are noted with spotty loss of hair.
Hair pulling	Persons may note that they habitually "touch" or pull at the involved area.	Fractured broken hairs in spotty distribution.
WIDESPREAD SCALP HAIR LOSS:		
Male pattern baldness	Usually a family history of baldness; adult onset.	Temporal baldness initially.
Following infection, surgery, childbirth or certain drugs (anticoagulants or cancer therapeutic agents)	Sudden and often total loss of hair is noticed.	Generalized hair loss without skin involvement or broken hairs.
Endocrine deficiency states (hypopituitarism or hypothryroidism)	Slowly progressive hair loss; loss of pubic and axillary hair often occurs in hypopituitarism. Hair thickening is more common in hypothyroidism.	Diminished axillary, pubic or lateral eyebrow hair; hair may become depigmented.

DIAGNOSTIC CONSIDERATIONS	HISTORY	PHYSICAL EXAM

HAIR EXCESS: (usually noted in females)

Endocrine abnormalities (adrenal or ovarian hyperfunction; adrenal steroid medication)	Acne and menstrual irregularity may be noted; muscles and voice may become more masculine.	Acne;(hypertrophy of the clitoris)
Unknown	Often a family history of the same problem.	The patient is often obese but otherwise normal.

Reference: Harrison's Principles of Internal Medicine. Seventh
     Edition. Pages 286-288.

HISTORY

Descriptors:

General descriptors: refer to inside cover.
Aggravating factors: trauma or laceration.
   Hand-wrist discomfort: worsened by pressure over the "funny bone", pronation of the forearm, exposure to the cold.
   Elbow-arm discomfort: worsened by lifting a cup or opening a door; exertion.

Associated Symptoms:

Weakness, numbness, swelling, pain or discoloration of the involved area; neck pain or other joint pains; chest pain; nausea, vomiting or sweating.

Medical History:

Rheumatoid arthritis; psoriasis; past trauma or fracture of the involved area; recent chest trauma or surgery; angina or myocardial infarction.

PHYSICAL EXAMINATION

Extremity: examine involved area for swelling, tenderness, discoloration, dislocation or deformity.
   Check strength of fingers, grip, wrist and upper arm.
   Check pinprick sensation in all fingers.
Special: If wrist or thumb pain, have the patient adduct the wrist while holding the thumb in his palm; percuss the "anatomical snuff box" at the base of the thumb; percuss the median nerves at the wrist.
   If the patient is over 40, press down on the head while the patient has his neck hyperextended, turned to the right and turned to the left. Does this maneuver reproduce the patient's discomfort.

GENERAL CONSIDERATIONS

Trauma, see TRAUMA.

Special considerations, see next page.

GENERAL CONSIDERATIONS
(Continued)

Special considerations for:

Hand trauma:
Wounds to the hand should always be carefully evaluated to
determine if there is any damage to the tendons, bones or
nerves. Punctures to the palmar fascia have a very high risk
of becoming infected. The injured hand should be elevated
to minimize swelling. Jewelry may irreversibly damage the
blood supply to the swollen hand; it should always be removed.

Wrist trauma:
It is safest to assume that tenderness in the "anatomical snuff
box" is a sign of a fracture of the navicular bone.

Pediatric trauma:
The upper extremity can be easily injured when children are
swung by the arms. Recurrent injury to the child, particularly
when it involves the upper extremities should be a clue that
the child may be suffering beatings (battered child syndrome).

Below are listed the diagnostic considerations for atraumatic
hand-wrist-arm problems based on the location of discomfort.

For shoulder pain, see JOINT EXTREMITY PAIN.

DIAGNOSTIC CONSIDERATIONS of atraumatic hand-wrist-arm problems based
on the location of discomfort.

USUAL LOCATION	COMMON DISEASE	FINDINGS
JOINT or SYNOVIUM DISEASE:		
Distal finger joints	Osteoarthritis	Multiple joint stiffness; mild deformity; bony enlargement of involved joints.

USUAL LOCATION	COMMON DISEASE	FINDINGS

JOINT or SYNOVIUM DISEASE:
(Continued)

Wrists, elbows, proximal finger joints	Rheumatoid arthritis	Multiple joint stiffness, swelling, tenderness; eventually marked deformity with ulnar deviation of hands and fingers, synovial thickening, nodules over extensor tendons and ulna.
Distal finger joints	Psoriatic arthritis	May mimic rheumatoid arthritis; psoriasis and finger nail destruction.
Elbow	"Bursitis"	Pain and swelling in posterior elbow.

TENDON - MUSCLE DISEASE

Tendons to thumb	Tenosynovitis; De Quervain's disease	Pain at base of thumb aggravated by movement of wrist or thumb; pain reproduced by flexing thumb, cupping in fingers, and flexing wrist in ulnar deviation.
3rd and 4th digits, palm	"Triggerfinger" Dupuytren's contracture	Catching or fixation of fingers in flexion; painless thickening of palmar fascia or tendon sheath.
Palmar aspect of fingers or hands	Infection	Often a preceding laceration; tender red swollen fingers and/or palm which may cause finger flexion, swelling and tenderness along tendon sheath and pain on attempted extension of fingers.
Elbows	Epicondylitis (tennis elbow)	Pain on opening doors, lifting a cup, playing tennis; tenderness over radial area of elbow.

USUAL LOCATION	COMMON DISEASE	FINDINGS
NERVE DISEASE:		Numbness, tingling and eventual weakness, which is:
Digits 1 - 3	Carpal tunnel syndrome	Worsened by forced flexion at wrist or tapping on carpal tunnel.
Digits 1 - 3 and thenar eminence	Pronator teres syndrome	Worsened by pronation of arm.
Digits 4 - 5	Ulnar syndrome	Worsened by pressure over ulnar nerve at "funny bone".
Several digits and contiguous areas of forearm	Cervical outlet	Worsened by cervical compression. Neck pain frequently noted.
VASCULAR DISEASE:		
Finger tips	Raynaud's phenomenon or disease	Fingers become painful and turn white then blue and red following exposure to cold.
REFERRED PAIN:		
Entire hand	Shoulder hand syndrome	Shoulder ache; hand burning; skin thickening, redness; joint stiffness and muscle atrophy. Usually follows intrathoracic injury (surgery, myocardial infarction).
Inner arm and shoulder	Angina, myocardial infarction	Angina: pain increasing with exertion, relieved by rest or nitroglycerin. Infarction: chest pain; nausea; vomiting; sweating.

HISTORY

Descriptors:

General descriptors: refer to inside cover.
Does the patient know events prior to the injury; does the
patient (particularly a child) seem normal to an observer
who knows the patient; was the patient unconscious--if so,
for how long.

Associated Symptoms:

Stupor; neck pain; motor or sensory changes; discharge from ear
or nose; seizure; loss of urine or bowel control or tongue
biting; other painful areas; lacerations.

Medical History:

Alcoholism; cardiovascular disease; epilepsy.

Medications:

Anticonvulsants; antihypertensive or antiarrhythmic drugs.

PHYSICAL EXAMINATION

Measure: blood pressure; pulse; respiration rate and pattern.
Mental status: orientation to time, place, person.
Head and neck: discoloration; palpable bony abnormalities;
  lacerations; point tenderness.
Ears: check tympanic membranes for discoloration.
Eyes: papilledema; equality of pupil size and reactivity to
  light.
Nose: clear discharge.
Neurological: cranial nerve function; deep tendon reflexes;
  plantar response; strength of extremities; sensation to pin
  prick.

GENERAL CONSIDERATIONS

If the patient complains of neck pain, neck fracture is possible.
Do not move the patient with severe neck pain or cervical spine
tenderness.

GENERAL CONSIDERATIONS:
   (Continued)

The patient is more likely to have suffered severe head trauma
(often associated with skull fracture) if any of the following
are present:

1. A history of unconsciousness for more than 5 minutes after
   the injury.
2. A history of not remembering events immediately prior to
   the injury.
3. A history of localized neurological abnormalities (excluding
   visual symptoms, e.g. transcient "flashes", blurred vision)
   following the trauma.
4. A physical examination that reveals: palpable bony malalignment of the skull; ear or nose discharge; ear drum discoloration; bilateral "black eyes"; localized neurological abnormalities. If the patient is stuporous, comatose or has abnormal respirations following trauma, severe injury is very
   likely.

When evaluating the patient with head trauma, one must also
consider the cause of the injury. Usually head injury precedes loss of consciousness. Rarely, however, the head may
be severely injured after a patient loses consciousness from
a convulsion or syncope attack. Careful questioning of witnesses
is therefore necessary.

Reference: Harrison's Principles of Internal Medicine. Seventh
           Edition. Pages 1764-1774.

HISTORY

Descriptors:

General descriptors: refer to inside cover.

Onset: does the headache awaken the patient from sleep; does it occur more often in the evening; chronic, recurrent or acute onset.

Location: unilateral or bilateral headaches; where does it seem to start. Is it primarily occipital.

Character: Pulsatile, tight (like a band around the head), or sharp.

Aggravating factors: head trauma; is the headache precipitated by anxiety, alcohol, certain foods or pressure over points of the head or face.

Past treatment or evaluation: skull x-ray; brain scan.

Associated Symptoms:

History of unconsciousness; change in memory or mentation; motor or sensory change; nausea; vomiting; stiff neck; fever; ear pain; eye pain; change in vision; nasal discharge or stuffy nose; muscle aches or pains; anxiety; depression; prodromata (flashing lights, "funny" feelings, preceding headache).

Medical History:

Any neurological disease; previous skull fracture; migraine headaches; emotional problems; sinus disease.

Medications:

Aspirin; codeine; ergot; caffeine; steroids; oral contraceptives; sedatives; decongestants; any injections.

Family History:

Headaches, especially migraine or cluster headaches.

PHYSICAL EXAMINATION

Measure: blood pressure; temperature.

Eyes: extraocular movements; pupil size and response to light; fundi: papilledema; retinal hemorrhages; check for absent venous pulsations.

PHYSICAL EXAMINATION
(Continued)

   Ears: bulging, perforation or inflammation of tympanic membrane.
   Sinus: check for sinus tenderness.
   Nose: discharge.
   Throat: tooth tenderness to percussion.
   Neck:stiffness.
   Neurological: examine cranial nerves, deep tendon and plantar
      reflexes.
   Special, if patient is over 40: Head: check temporal arteries
      for tenderness; observe if pressure on the head while the
      patient has his neck hyperextended, turned to the right and
      turned to the left reproduces or exacerbates the headache.
   Eyes: check visual fields.

GENERAL CONSIDERATIONS
   Headache is most often due to noxious stimulation of the inter-
   cranial vessels or membranes, the cranial or cervical nerves or
   the cranial or cervical muscles. The brain itself is pain in-
   sensitive.

   The vast majority of headaches in all age groups are "muscle
   tension", "vascular" or those associated with febrile or viral
   illnesses.

DIAGNOSTIC CONSIDERATIONS	HISTORY	PHYSICAL EXAM
MUSCLE TENSION HEADACHES:		
	Constant bandlike pressure lasting days to weeks; usually worse at the end of the day; often occipital location; anxiety may cause or worsen the attack.	May reveal muscular tension in the neck.
VASCULAR HEADACHES:		
Classic migraine	Throbbing, often unilateral frontal headache lasting several days; visual prodromata, nausea and vomiting often preceed the attack; (continued on next page)	Neurological abnormalities may rarely be noted during an attack; usually normal.

DIAGNOSTIC CONSIDERATIONS	HISTORY	PHYSICAL EXAM
VASCULAR HEADACHES: (Continued)		
Classic migraine (Continued)	(Continued) family history of migraine frequently noted; may be caused by alcohol or stress.	See preceeding page.
Common migraine	Character of headache and prodromata usually less clearly defined than in classic migraine; family history uncommon.	Normal.
Cluster headaches	Brief frontal headaches most often noted at night; associated with tearing and nasal stuffiness; occur in "clusters" with many months symptom-free.	Tearing and nasal discharge may be present.
SINUS HEADACHE:	Frontal or maxillary pain often associated with nasal stuffiness and discharge.	Sinus tenderness and nasal discharge are usually present; tooth tenderness to percussion.
NON-SPECIFIC HEADACHE:		
(With febrile or viral illness)	Muscle aches and pains; cough; sore throat often noted.	Mild temperature elevation may be present.
CERVICAL ARTHRITIS	Occipital and neck ache may be worse with neck movement; patient usually over 40 years of age.	Cervical compression often reproduces or worsens the pain; decreased reflexes in the arms may rarely be present.

DIAGNOSTIC CONSIDERATIONS	HISTORY	PHYSICAL EXAM
TRIGEMINAL NEURALGIA	Brief jabs of facial pain often caused by touching a "trigger point".	Touching certain areas of the face may cause the pain.

RARE BUT EXTREMELY SERIOUS CAUSES OF HEADACHE:

Meningitis	Recent development of fever, headache, nausea and vomiting.	Fever; stiff neck; occasional cranial nerve abnormalities.
Subarachnoid bleeding	Very rapid onset of unilateral headache often with change in consciousness or neurological function; vomiting is common.	Blood pressure frequently elevated; stiff neck; occasional cranial nerve abnormalities.
Temporal arteritis	Temporal headaches often with generalized chronic muscle aches and weakness in the patient over 40 years of age; transcient decreases in vision may progress to blindness.	Temporal artery tenderness and abnormal visual fields may be present.
Malignant hypertension	Blurring vision; a history of hypertension is common.	Diastolic blood pressure usually more than 130 mm of mercury; fundoscopy may reveal exudates , papilledema and hemorrhages.
Intracranial mass (abscess, tumor)	No characteristic history; most suspect is the recent development of a headache that does not fit the above patterns.	Focal neurological abnormalities; absent venous pulsations or papilledema may be noted.

DIAGNOSTIC CONSIDERATIONS	HISTORY	PHYSICAL EXAM

RARE BUT EXTREMELY SERIOUS CAUSES OF HEADACHE:
(Continued)

Subdural hematoma	Headache and level of consciousness may wax and wane over months; usually in alcoholics who have sustained moderate head injury.	Usually is normal though neurological abnormalities may be present.

Reference: Harrison's Principles of Internal Medicine. Seventh
         Edition. Pages 18-24.

HISTORY

Descriptors:

General descriptors: refer to inside cover.
How long was patient in hot environment; how warm was the
environment; what was patient doing in it.
Past treatment or evaluation: if the patient's temperature
was taken, what was it.

Associated Symptoms:
Headache; change in mentation; loss of consciousness; nausea;
vomiting; diarrhea; decreased urine output; sweating; cold
skin; muscle cramps; bleeding from any site.

Medical History:
Alcoholism; heart disease; hypertension; diabetes.

Medications:
Alcohol; antihypertensive medication; diuretics; atropine
medications; benztropin(Cogentin), phenothiazine tranquilizers.

PHYSICAL EXAMINATION

Measure: rectal temperature; respiratory rate; blood pressure
and pulse lying and sitting.
Skin: is sweating present or absent; skin color and warmth.
Neurological: cranial nerves; deep tendon reflexes and plantar
response.

GENERAL CONSIDERATIONS

Collapse during hot weather may be due to a mild disease manifested by faintness, cold clammy skin and minimal temperature
elevation for which little treatment is required (heat prostra-
tion).

On the other hand, in true heat stroke the patient may be comatose or delirious; the physical examination often reveals a

GENERAL CONSIDERATIONS
(Continued)

temperature more than 103 degrees and hot dry skin. Heroic
prompt treatment is required to avoid death or irreversible
brain damage.

Heat stroke occurs more commonly under conditions which pre-
dispose to dehydration (antihypertensive medication and alcohol)
or cause an inability to sweat adequately (excessive clothing,
excessive exercise, anticholinergic medications, benztropin,
phenothiazines, diabetes, atherosclerosis or old age).

Reference: Harrison's Principles of Internal Medicine.   Seventh
Edition.   Pages 51-52.

HISTORY

Descriptors:

General descriptors: refer to inside cover.
  Is hernia always present or present only under certain
  circumstances; is it reducible.
Location: apparent size, one or both sides.
Past evaluation: has presence of hernia ever been confirmed
  by a physician; if so, when.

Associated Symptoms:
Scrotal mass; change in bowel habits; abdominal pain or distension; need to strain to move bowels or urinate; recent onset
of cough or change in chronic cough.

PHYSICAL EXAMINATION

Genital: examine hernia and testes.
Rectal: stool for occult blood; check prostate size.

GENERAL CONSIDERATIONS

The appearance of an inguinal hernia in the patient over age
50 should make the examiner consider causes for periodic
increases in intra-abdominal pressure which could be contri-
buting to the development of a hernia.

Diseases that could cause increased intra-abdominal pressure
include prostate disease causing urethral obstruction, pulmonary disease with cough, and large bowel malignancy causing
partial bowel obstruction.

In children the presence of one hernia may indicate bilateral
weakness of the inguinal canal. Hydrocoeles (smooth scrotal
masses that transilluminate) are common in the first year of
life and may be confused with an irreducible inguinal hernia.

HISTORY

Descriptors:

> General descriptors: refer to inside cover.
> Aggravating factors: did hiccough begin after rapid eating.

Associated Symptoms:
Abdominal pain; weakness; chest pain; new cough or change in cough pattern; trouble swallowing; anxiety.

Medical History:
Alcoholism; kidney, liver or neurological disease.

PHYSICAL EXAMINATION

Abdomen: tenderness; masses; distension.

GENERAL CONSIDERATIONS

Hiccough is an involuntary inspiratory movement of the diaphragm followed by closure of the glottis. It is only significant when persistent.

Persistent hiccoughs may be caused by stimulation of the phrenic nerve due to abdominal disease (particularly gastritis or gastric distention), intra-thoracic processes impinging on the phrenic nerve (lung tumor), or neurological disease. Renal failure and encephalitis are frequent causes of persistent hiccough.

Transcient hiccoughs occur in normal individuals often following rapid eating.

HISTORY

Descriptors:

General descriptors: refer to inside cover.

ACUTE
(onset less than 2 weeks ago)

Associated Symptoms:
Cough; fever; sore throat; trouble breathing; wheezing.

PHYSICAL EXAMINATION

Measure: temperature
Throat: (do not use instrument examination in a child with drooling or stridor); erythema.

CHRONIC
(onset gradual or noted more than two weeks ago).

Associated Symptoms:
Weight loss, cough, hemoptysis; neck or chest pain; trouble swallowing or moving; change in sensation; thickening of hair or cold intolerance.

Medical History
Any chronic disease particularly thyroid or neurological diseases. Alcoholism.

Environmental History:
Is patient a smoker, drinker or singer.

PHYSICAL EXAMINATION

Throat: Laryngoscopy: Vocal cord movement; masses.
Neck: Tracheal deviation, neck mass.
Skin: Coarse hair; thickened skin.
Neurological:
  Achilles Reflex - delayed relaxation phase.

GENERAL CONSIDERATIONS

The commonest cause for acute hoarseness is laryngitis in which the patient usually has symptoms of a cold and often has a sore throat. The child, particularly from ages three to seven, who is hoarse may have epiglottitis, a life threatening condition characterized by trouble breathing, drooling, sore throat and respiratory stridor.

Hoarseness which persists for more than two weeks will require laryngoscopic evaluation. Considerations for chronic hoarseness are listed below. A "hoarse" voice in boys at puberty is normal and requires no evaluation.

DIAGNOSTIC CONSIDERATIONS	HISTORY	PHYSICAL EXAM
"myxomatous degeneration" or chronic inflammation.	Patient is usually a smoker and drinker. Problem persists for years and causes a husky voice.	Myxomatous degeneration, thickening or inflammation of vocal cords.
Tumor of the vocal cord.	Progressive hoarseness in the smoker and drinker.	Tumor of the cord noted.
Laryngeal nerve paralysis	Progressive hoarseness; weight loss. cough or hemoptysis may also be noted due to tumor in the lung. Rarely associated with cerebrovascular disease.	Poor movement of a vocal cord.
Hypothyroidism	Slowly progressive hoarseness; thickened skin, cold intolerance.	Coarse hair; slow relaxation of deep tendon reflexes; normal vocal cords.

Reference: Harrison's Principles of Internal Medicine. Seventh Edition. Page 1274.

HISTORY

Descriptors:

General descriptors: refer to inside cover.
Aggravating factors: was hyperactivity preceded by a birth, death or separation in the family; is the hyperactivity worse when the child is surrounded by other children or placed in a new environment; does the family speak a foreign language at home.
Past treatment or evaluation: has the child had psychological tests or a trial of medication in the past.

Associated Symptoms:

Trouble seeing, hearing or speaking; "clumsiness"; labile moods; learning problems; seizures.

Medical History:

Mental retardation; seizure disorder; severe birth trauma or neonatal jaundice.

Medications:

Barbiturates; tranquilizers; amphetamines (Ritalin).

PHYSICAL EXAMINATION

Measure: weight; height; head circumference.
General: observe the "activity" of the child in the examining room; are the child's movements clumsy; are there tremors or uncontrolled movements of the extremities; is the child's mood labile.
Ears: check hearing.
Eyes: check visual acuity.
Neck: check for thyroid enlargement.
Neurological: check developmental milestones appropriate for the child's age.
   Cranial nerve examination.
   Deep tendon reflexes and plantar reflex.
   Have the child perform rapid rhythmic movements such as clapping the hands, jumping on one foot.

GENERAL CONSIDERATIONS

Hyperactivity is a common symptom that should not be confused with the syndrome of hyperkinesis or minimal brain dysfunction. Hyperactivity is an extremely subjective complaint made by parents and teachers about children. It is a symptom, not a diagnosis.

Common causes for hyperactivity include: most normal children (especially ages 2 - 4); older children of above average intelligence and inquisitive behavior; children reacting to external problems in school, at home, with friends or siblings; a child's inability to adjust to different standards of behavior and performance expected at home and in school; children who do not speak English in schools which are not bilingual; hearing difficulties; drug reactions; visual difficulties. Other causes of hyperactivity include: seizure disorders; retardation; hyperthyroidism and psychiatric disorders.

The hyperkinesis syndrome consists of hyperactivity and easy distractability, labile moods, poor impulse control, explosive moods and learning problems. The hyperkinesis syndrome may be part of the minimal brain dysfunction syndrome.

Minimal brain dysfunction is seen in the "clumsy" child who is usually of average intelligence and can perform normal neurological functions for his age. Fine coordination, however, often demonstrates abnormalities of function.

HISTORY

Descriptors:

General descriptors: refer to inside cover.
Onset: age at which elevated blood pressure was first observed.
Precipitating/aggravating factors: concurrent ingestion of
  adrenal steroids, oral contraceptives, decongestants or bronchodilators; is patient pregnant.
Past evaluation or treatment: last urinalysis or intravenous
  pyelogram; what have been past blood pressure values.

Associated Symptoms:

Blood in urine; pain on urination or polyuria; chest pain;
foot or ankle swelling; spells of pallor, dyspnea, sweating and
nervousness; faintness upon sudden standing.

Medical History:

Kidney disease; cardiovascular disease; diabetes; toxemia
of pregnancy.

Medications:

Digitalis; diuretics; blood pressure medication.

Family History:

Hypertension; kidney disease; cardiovascular disease; diabetes.

False Positive:

"High blood pressure" or "hypertension" often is used by patients
to describe feelings of anxiety.
 Decongestants may cause transient blood pressure elevation.

PHYSICAL EXAMINATION

Measure: weight; pulse rate; blood pressure lying and standing
  in both arms.

Eyes, fundi: arteriovenous ratio; focal constrictions; hemorrhages; exudates; papilledema.

PHYSICAL EXAMINATION
(Continued)

Chest: rales.
Cardiac: gallops; murmurs; apical impulse prolonged through
more than one half of systole or felt in more than one rib
interspace.
Abdomen: truncal obesity; renal masses; flank bruits.
Pulses: carotid bruit; delay in femoral pulse relative to radial
pulse; diminished pulses.
Skin: stria; plethoric facies; hirsutism.

GENERAL CONSIDERATIONS

Patients with persistently elevated blood pressure risk
damage to certain organs of their body (so-called "end-
organs"). Evidence of "end-organ" damage in the hypertensive patient constitutes a strong indication for immediate therapy. In less than 20% of hypertensive patients
a specific disease is identified as the cause of hypertension; cure of the disease often cures the hypertension.

The cause of hypertension is usually unknown (essential
hypertension).

Listed below are the diseases which may cause hypertension
and the common end organ changes of hypertension.

DIAGNOSTIC CONSIDERATIONS	HISTORY	PHYSICAL EXAM
SECONDARY CAUSES OF HYPERTENSION:		
Renal vascular disease	Hypertension of recent onset in a young female or person past the age of 50.	Bruit may be heard in the flanks.

DIAGNOSTIC CONSIDERATIONS	HISTORY	PHYSICAL EXAM
SECONDARY CAUSES OF HYPERTENSION: (Continued)		
Aldosterone secreting tumor	Weakness; polyuria. Often asymptomatic.	Usually normal.
Renal disease	History of renal disease; hematuria.	Usually normal; rarely a renal mass is palpable.
Coarctation of aorta	Usually young patients.	Delay in femoral pulse relative to radial pulse.
Pheochromo-cytoma	Spells of sweating, blanching and anxiety.	Orthostatic hypo-tension.
Cushing's disease	Weakness; obesity.	Truncal obesity; hirsutism, stria and plethoric facies.
Medication-related	Oral contraceptives; adrenal steroids; de-congestants; broncho-dilators.	Normal (or reflecting the disease for which medication is being given).
Toxemia of pregnancy	Ankle swelling; patient usually more than 6 months pregnant.	Pregnant female.
END ORGAN EFFECTS OF HYPERTENSION:		
Athero-sclerosis	Angina pectoris; myocar-dial infarction; cere-brovascular accident.	Usually hypertensive retinopathy (see below); carotid bruit or de-creased pulses.

DIAGNOSTIC CONSIDERATIONS	HISTORY	PHYSICAL EXAM
END ORGAN EFFECTS OF HYPERTENSION: (Continued)		
Heart enlargement or failure	Dyspnea; orthopnea; paroxysmal nocturnal dyspnea; ankle edema.	Prolonged or enlarged apical impulse; third or fourth heart sound; edema; rales.
Hypertensive retinopathy	Change in vision occurs uncommonly.	Arteriovenous ratio less than 1 to 2; arteriovenous "nicking"; hemorrhages, exudates or papilledema.
Renal failure		Hypertensive retinopathy.

Reference: Harrison's Principles of Internal Medicine. Seventh Edition. Pages 188-191.

HISTORY

Descriptors:

General descriptors: refer to inside cover. Specify exact
nature of complaint and location of discomfort (if any).
Aggravating factors: relation of complaint to bowel movements,
meals, position, foods (liquids, solids, milk).
Relieving factors: relief by antacids, belching.
Past treatment or evaluation: past X-ray (barium swallow or
barium enema; gall bladder x-ray).

Associated Symptoms:

Abdominal pain; nausea and vomiting; change in bowel habits;
black stools; measured change in abdominal girth; greasy bowel
movements; weight change; flatulence; belching; regurgitation;
anxiety or depression.

Medical History:

Abdominal surgery; ulcer disease; colitis; diverticulosis;
alcoholism; liver disease; hiatus hernia; obesity; emotional
problems.

Medications:

Diuretics ; antidepressants; tranquilizers; antacids; "antispasmodics" (Librax, belladonna).

PHYSICAL EXAMINATION

Measure: weigh patient.
Abdomen: masses; tenderness; tympany; bowel sounds.
Rectal: stool occult blood.

GENERAL CONSIDERATIONS

When associated with abdominal pain, the location and character
of the pain are important clues to the possible cause of "indigestion"   (See ABDOMINAL PAIN). Otherwise, indigestion is
often an indistinct entity which may be caused by any of the
diseases listed with ABDOMINAL PAIN as well as the following:

DIAGNOSTIC CONSIDERATIONS	HISTORY	PHYSICAL EXAM
Aerophagia/Flat-ulence (bloating, belching and gas)	Chronic history; often worsened by certain foods. No other change in health status.	Occasional mild diffuse abdominal distention and hyperresonance. No weight change.

DIAGNOSTIC CONSIDERATIONS	HISTORY	PHYSICAL EXAM
Maldigestion, Malabsorption or food intolerance	Certain foods may cause diarrhea; greasy bowel movements are noted occasionally; weight loss may be noted.	Weight loss may be present.
Gastrointestinal Pathology (see also AB-DOMINAL PAIN)	Weight loss or abdominal pain; change in bowel habits; nausea or vomiting is frequently noted.	Abdominal masses; tenderness or stool positive for occult blood are frequently present.
Bloating (abdominal swelling)		
Ascites	Often a history of alcoholism, liver disease and a protuberant abdomen.	Ascites and spider angiomata are noted.
Obesity	Obesity.	Obesity.
Aerophagia/ Flatulence	See above.	See above.
Colic (newborns and infants)	Brief paroxysms of crying and writhing often relieved by passing gas.	Increased bowel sounds during the attack.
"Functional Abdominal Complaints"	Often recurrent chronic and nondescript complaints resulting in no demonstrable health changes to the patient. Depression and a history of emotional disease are occasionally noted.	Repeatedly normal examinations.

Reference: Harrison's Principles of Internal Medicine. 7th edition, Pages 208-210.

HISTORY

Descriptors:

General descriptors: refer to inside cover.
Fertility of patient or spouse in other marriages; how long
has the patient been trying to have children; has the patient
used contraceptives: when and for how long.
Past treatment or evaluation: extent of evaluation: semen
  analysis (if male); pelvic examination, basal temperature
  analysis (if female).

Associated Symptoms:

Male: Failure of erection; testicular pain or swelling.
Female: Vaginal discharge; abdominal or pelvic pain; pain on
  intercourse; irregular menses.

Medical History:

Abdominal/Pelvic surgery; emotional problems.
Male: mumps.
Female: endometriosis; past pregnancies or abortions.
  Venereal disease.

Environmental History:

Excessive or prolonged exposure to x-rays, chemicals or oral
contraceptives.

PHYSICAL EXAMINATION

Genital: male-testes for size; penis for hypospadias.
          female-pelvic masses or tenderness.
Skin: note distribution of body hair. Is it appropriate for
  the sex of the patient.

GENERAL CONSIDERATIONS

Infertility may be the result of many factors. Male fertility
may be inadequate due to poor sexual performance of the male
or decreased viability, amount or quality of the sperm. Female
fertility requires adequate ovulation and function of the
fallopian tubes, cervix and uterus. Either sex may become in-
fertile due to emotional stress, external factors (irradiation,
etc.) or inadequate hormonal function.

Reference: Harrison's Principles of Internal Medicine. 7th edition,
            Pages 249-251.

HISTORY

Descriptors:

Ceneral descriptors: refer to inside cover.
Onset: note carefully when first symptoms were noted.
Aggravating factors: Hepatotoxic medications: isoniazid;
phenothiazines; oral contraceptives; Halothane anesthesia;
methyl-dopa.

Hepatotoxic substances:intravenous narcotics; alcohol;
chemical solvents; exposure or injection of blood serum
in the past 6 months.

Hemolytic medications: sulfa drugs; nitrofurantoin;
quinidine.

Past treatment or evaluation: what, if any, tests have been
done for the problem; has a liver biopsy been performed.

Associated Symptoms:

Headache; loss of appetite; nausea; vomiting; fever, shaking
chills; abdominal pain; change in weight; abdominal
swelling; black, tarry or bloody bowel movements; light
stools; dark urine; change in mentation; joint pain; pruritis

Medical History:

Alcoholism; gallstones; liver disease (cirrhosis); past
gastrointestinal bleeding; drug addiction; mononucleosis;
blood disease; history of malignancy.

Medications:

Any; see Aggravating factors above.

Family History:

Jaundice.

Environmental History:

Has the patient had any close contact with jaundiced persons;
work with solvents; nature of water supply; foreign travel in
the past 6 months.

PHYSICAL EXAMINATION

Measure: blood pressure; pulse; temperature.
Mental status: is patient aware of his surroundings, the
   date and recent events.
Abdomen: check for ascites; liver or spleen size; masses or
   tenderness.
Rectal: stool for occult blood.
Genital, male: check for testicle size and gynecomastia.
Skin: spider angiomata; needle tracts; palmar erythema.
Nodes: enlargement.
Extremities: have the patient hold his arms in front of him
   with wrists hyperextended. Is a flapping movement noted.

GENERAL CONSIDERATIONS

Neonate:
In the neonate the major helpful characteristic is the time
of appearance of jaundice. That appearing within the first
24 hours of birth or after the 4th day usually indicates
severe hemolysis in the former instance and any of the adult
considerations (see below) or severe infection in the latter.

Jaundice appearing from the 2nd to 4th day after birth is
usually benign and self-limited unless it persists longer
than 1 week from onset. Persistence may indicate biliary
atresia, hypothyroidism, hepatitis or hemolysis.

Pediatric and adult:
Jaundice is caused by the excessive accumulation of blood
breakdown products (bilirubin) in the body. Excessive
bilirubin production secondary to hemolysis may cause jaundice. Jaundice may also be caused by inadequate transport,
conjugation, metabolism or excrection of normal bilirubin
loads by an inadequate hepatobiliary system.

Disorders of transport and conjugation (Dubin-Rotor and Gilbert
Syndromes) as well as chronic hemolytic states often cause
elevated serum bilirubin levels that are not detected by
physical examination and the patient usually feels well. On
the other hand, even when the patient feels poorly from
liver diseases such as hepatitis or that due to infiltrating
carcinoma,liver function abnormalities are discovered only by
laboratory analysis.

GENERAL CONSIDERATIONS
(Continued)

Therefore the realistic evaluation of jaundice and liver
disease often depends on serial determinations of liver
function tests since the history and physical examination
may seem deceptively "normal". Clinical evaluation may
be helpful in differentiating the causes of jaundice listed
below.

DIAGNOSTIC CONSIDERATIONS	HISTORY	PHYSICAL EXAM
Viral hepatitis (serum hepatitis, infectious hepatitis, mononucleosis)	Onset of jaundice over days or weeks; right upper quadrant discomfort; nausea and vomiting; arthralgias, fever and headache; dark urine and light stools are frequently noted; a history of contact with blood products, others with jaundice or a fecally contaminated water supply may be obtained; the patient may be a drug addict.	Jaundice; large tender liver; fever; lymphadenopathy and needle tracts may be present.
Toxic hepatitis: alcohol, drugs (Halothane, methyldopa, isoniazid, phenothiazines, oral contraceptives), chemical solvents.	Onset of jaundice over days or weeks; history of ingestion of medications, solvents or excessive alcohol; dark urine, light stools and right upper quadrant discomfort may be noted.	Jaundice; large tender liver occasionally.

DIAGNOSTIC CONSIDERATIONS	HISTORY	PHYSICAL EXAM
Obstruction of biliary flow	Symptoms may be acute or chronic; jaundice; pruritis; light stools and dark urine are frequently noted; a history of gallstones may be present.	Jaundice; the gall bladder may be palpable whereas the liver is often normal size.
Chronic liver disease (cirrhosis)	Chronic jaundice; patient may have a history of any of the causes of jaundice listed above.	Jaundice; spider angiomata; palmar erythema; splenomegaly; periperal edema; ascites; the liver is often not palpable; males may have gynecomastia and small soft testicles.
Liver failure	Most often the patient with chronic liver disease suffers gastrointestinal bleeding, infection or repeated liver insult (e.g. alcoholic binge) leading to disorientation, stupor and coma.	Usually the above signs of chronic liver disease are present; a flapping movement of the extended arms, stupor or coma are common.

Reference: Harrison's Principles of Internal Medicine. Seventh Edition. Pages 221-227.

HISTORY

Descriptors:

General descriptors: refer to inside cover.
Is pain in joints, muscles or both.
If joint pain: is the pain localized to one joint or many;
  has the pain stayed in the same joint or has it been
  migratory.
If one area only is involved: ask the specific questions
  below before proceeding to the general evaluation.

REGIONAL JOINT AND EXTREMITY COMPLAINTS:

Hand-wrist-arm pain: see HAND-WRIST-ARM PROBLEMS.

Shoulder pain - left arm pain (in adults only):
    Aggravating factors: pain worsened or brought on by exercise;
    does movement of shoulder aggravate pain.
    Associated symptoms: chest pain.
    Medical history: diabetes; hypertension; cardiovascular
    disease; past shoulder dislocations or episodes of bursitis.

Hip pain:
    Associated symptoms: inability to walk; low back pain.
    Medical history: sickle cell disease; past surgery on or
    near hip.

Knee pain:
    Associated symptoms: feeling of snapping, catching or buckling;
    pain on squatting or running up and down stairs; hip pain.
    Medical history: hemophilia; past knee trauma or surgery.

Calf pain - leg pain (in adults only):
    Aggravating factors: pain only on exertion, relieved by rest;
    did pain follow trauma.
    Associated symptoms: calf swelling or tenderness; low back
    pain; pain worsened by coughing.
    Medical history: cardiovascular disease; chronic lung disease;
    recent surgery or prolonged immobilization; thrombophlebitis.
    Medications: oral contraceptives.

Foot - ankle pain: see FOOT-ANKLE PAIN.

GENERALIZED JOINT AND EXTREMITY PAIN

General Descriptors: is the pain worse toward the end of the
    day; have the joint complaints been present for 6 weeks or
    longer.

Associated Symptoms:
    Fever; stiffness of joints in morning (how long); skin lesions;
    back pain; cough; runny nose; diarrhea; headache; finger pain
    and discoloration in the cold.

Medical History:
    Rheumatoid arthritis; gout; gonorrhea; past trauma or surgery
    to involved area; rheumatic fever; penile or vaginal discharge.

Environmental:
    Recent epidemic of streptococcal pharyngitis.

PHYSICAL EXAMINATION

    Measure: temperature.
    Extremity joint: swelling; tenderness; deformity; discoloration
      or warmth; test range of motion.
      If any of below involved:
        Knee: check hip range of motion; point tenderness of
          knee; tests of stability of knee joint by:
          1. With the patient lying on his back and knee flexed,
             the examiner pushes and pulls just below the knee
             (examiner's fingers are in popliteal fossa) to test
             for anteroposterior glide of the knee.
          2. With the patient on his abdomen and with the knee
             flexed, the examiner rotates the leg while pressing
             down on the leg and repeats the rotation while
             pulling up on the leg.

    Shoulder: point tenderness.

    Calf: tenderness to palpation; pain on dorsiflexion of
      the foot; difference in calf size; are superficial veins
      dilated on the involved side.

    Leg: does straight leg raising reproduce leg pain; hip
      range of motion.

GENERALIZED JOINT COMPLAINTS

DIAGNOSTIC CONSIDERATIONS	HISTORY	PHYSICAL EXAM
Degenerative joint disease (osteoarthritis)	Persistent joint pains; one or more joints involved; uncommon before age 40; seldom afflicts wrists, elbows or shoulders; development is accelerated in previously injured joint.	Involved joint usually not hot; effusion rare; synovial thickening is rare; Heberden's nodes and bony joint enlargement and deformity may occur.
Nonspecific or the arthralgia often associated with viral infections (upper respiratory illness, etc.)	Acute polyarthralgias are often associated with "flu"-like symptoms; chronic nonspecific arthralgias often "work out" in several minutes.	No joint abnormalities.
Infective (gonococcus, staphylococcal, hemophilus)	One or more joints; any age; slower onset than gout; often history of gonococcal exposure or infection, urethral or vaginal discharge.	Effusions common; fever; skin rashes; warm, tender, swollen joint(s).
Crystal-induced (gout; pseudo-gout)	One or more joints; male; metatarsal-phalangeal joint of big toe eventually affected in 90% cases of gout; sudden attacks; history of hyperuricemia or previous attack of gout; family history of gout.	Warm, red, tender swollen joints (Tophi may be present).

GENERALIZED JOINT COMPLAINTS
(Continued)

DIAGNOSTIC CONSIDERATIONS	HISTORY	PHYSICAL EXAM
Rheumatoid arthritis	Joint pain lasting more than 6 weeks; morning joint stiffness.	Pain on motion or tenderness of at least one joint; effusion or soft tissue swelling of one or more joints; joint involvement usually symmetrical; subcutaneous nodules on extensor surfaces of extremities;(eventual joint deformity is common).
Connective tissue disease	Finger pain and discoloration in the cold (Raynaud's phenomenon) may be noted.	Persistant skin rashes may be present; no joint deformity.

CONSIDERATIONS FOR REGIONAL JOINT EXTREMITY COMPLAINTS

DIAGNOSTIC CONSIDERATIONS	HISTORY	PHYSICAL EXAM
Pain primarily limited to a bone (extra-articular and extramuscular)		
Fracture or dislocation	Trauma; inability of the injured area to function normally. Note: upper extremity injury in children may be part of the 'battered child syndrome.'	Displacement, deformity or unusual mobility of the involved area; tenderness and swelling are frequently present.

CONSIDERATIONS FOR REGIONAL JOINT EXTREMITY COMPLAINTS
(Continued)

DIAGNOSTIC CONSIDERATIONS	HISTORY	PHYSICAL EXAM
Pain primarily limited to a bone (extra-articular and extramuscular) (Continued)		
Bone infection (Osteomyelitis)	Bone pain; fever; limp.	Fever; bone tenderness; warmth and induration of the overlying skin.
Knee pain only, adult:		
Meniscus or ligament tears	Catching or buckling of the knee.	Point tenderness over the knee ligaments or cartilage; occasional knee instability.
Referred pain from hip	Hip pain.	Hip pain; abnormal hip range of motion.
Knee pain only, pediatric: see also hip pain below since hip disease often refers pain to the knee in children.		
Hemophilia	Effusion following minimal trauma; family history of bleeding may be noted.	Joint effusion or swelling.
Schlatter's disease	Pain on squatting.	Tenderness over the tibial tuberosities.
Chondromalacia patella	Pain on running up or descending stairs.	Tenderness on compressing the patella.
Hip pain only:		
Osteoarthritis (adult)	Hip pain; limping; age usually over 50 years.	Abnormal range of motion of hip.
Legg-Perthes disease or slipped femoral epiphysis (pediatric)	Hip pain or knee pain; limping.	Abnormal range of motion of hip.

CONSIDERATIONS FOR REGIONAL JOINT EXTREMITY COMPLAINTS
                        (Continued)

DIAGNOSTIC CONSIDERATIONS	HISTORY	PHYSICAL EXAM
Hip pain only: (Continued)		
Necrosis of hip (any age)	Patient taking adrenal steroids or patient with sickle cell disease; hip pain.	Abnormal hip range of motion.
Shoulder pain only:		
Angina	Substernal chest and arm pain usually present; pain usually caused by exertion and relieved by rest or nitroglycerin.	Shoulder examination normal.
Bursitis (supraspinatus or bicipital bursa)	Pain on shoulder movement, particularly on combing hair (supraspinatus) or lifting (bicipital).	Point tenderness, swelling and warmth of the shoulder may be present.

Hand, arm pain only: see HAND, WRIST, ARM PROBLEMS.

Foot, ankle pain only: see FOOT, ANKLE PROBLEMS.

Calf or leg pain, numbness or tingling only (generally adults):

Referred pain (Sciatica)	Low back pain; leg pain or numbness worse with coughing.	Straight leg raising past 60 degrees increases discomfort in back or leg.
Arterial disease (acute embolus)	Patients often have a history of heart disease; acute pain eventually leading to paresthesias and to paralysis.	Pallor and absent pulse in the involved extremity.

CONSIDERATIONS FOR REGIONAL JOINT EXTREMITY COMPLAINTS
(Continued)

DIAGNOSTIC CONSIDERATIONS	HISTORY	PHYSICAL EXAM

Calf or leg pain, numbness or tingling only (generally adults): (Continued)

Arterial disease (chronic claudication)	Patient complains of pain, cramp or fatigue with exercise and notes relief with rest.	Skin atrophy; decreased pulses; decreased hair growth and "heaped up" nails may be present.
Venous Diseases:		
Venous thrombosis	Aching, tenderness, swelling of leg; often symptoms are minimal; rarely clots from the legs may embolize to the lungs causing chest pain, dyspnea and hemoptysis (pulmonary embolus).	On the involved side: dorsiflexion of the foot often causes pain (Homan's sign); tenderness may be noted along the thrombosed vein; swelling of the calf and dilation of the superficial veins are frequently present.
Venous insufficiency	Chronic aching or heaviness in the leg(s); elevation of the limb relieves pain.	Dilated varicose veins; edema, brawny induration and brown discoloration of the skin are frequently present.
Muscle "strain"	Usually a history of excessive exertion (followed by bilateral dull ache in calves or thighs).	Usually normal; mild muscle tenderness may be present.

Reference: Harrison's Principles of Internal Medicine. Seventh Edition. Pages 1984-2015.

HISTORY

Descriptors:

General descriptors: refer to inside cover.
Aggravating factors: how much can the patient do before feeling
    tired; are there family, job or school problems; is the
    tiredness only noted during exertion.

Associated Symptoms:

Depression or anxiety; tiredness on arising in the morning;
trouble concentrating; lack of interest in sex; decreased
appetite; weight loss; change in bowel habits; fever or chills;
sore throat; new or unusual cough; breathing trouble; headache;
chest or abdominal pain; muscle weakness; excessive sleeping.

Medical History:

Emotional disease; any chronic diseases.

Medications:

Any; particularly methyl-dopa (aldomet) or reserpine; sedatives;
tranquilizers; antidepressants; antihistamines.

PHYSICAL EXAMINATION

Measure: blood pressure; pulse; temperature; weight.
Throat: erythema.
Heart: murmurs; rubs; gallops.
Chest: any abnormalities.
Abdomen: masses or tenderness.
Nodes: lymphadenopathy.
Pediatric: neck for stiffness; fontanels for bulging.

NOTE: Does the patient require stimulation to stay awake.

GENERAL CONSIDERATIONS

In the adult the most common cause of lethargy or being "tired
out" is depression, which usually is situational in nature and
treatable. Typical associated symptoms include: feeling tired
on arising in the morning; small tasks seeming like large obstacles;
emotional lability; trouble concentrating; multiple aches and pains;
lack of interest in sex; change in appetite and bowel patterns; inability to sleep. The physical examination is normal and careful

GENERAL CONSIDERATIONS
(Continued)

history of the patient's personal life will often reveal obvious reasons for the depression.

Lethargy may also be the nonspecific manifestation of numerous underlying diseases. Acute diseases, particularly those associated with fever or cerebral dysfunction (upper respiratory infection, mononucleosis, meningitis, etc.) often have associated fatigue and lethargy.

Chronic diseases, particularly anemia, cardiorespiratory failure and low grade infections (endocarditis, urinary tract infections, tuberculosis) cause lethargy.

Side effects of the drugs listed may include depression and/or lethargy.

The lethargic child is usually suffering from one of the acute or chronic causes listed above. Depression is rarely a cause of lethargy in the pediatric age group.

NOTE. The person who requires stimulation to remain awake is stuporous. (See UNCONSCIOUS (stupor)).

Reference: Harrison's Principles of Internal Medicine. Seventh Edition. Pages 68-72.

HISTORY

Descriptors:

General descriptors: refer to inside cover.

It is often more revealing to examine the lesion before obtaining any history. The nature of the lesion may be obvious from examination.

Location: Aggravating factors:
Cervical node region: recent sore throat; dental problems; gum problems; pharyngitis; scalp wounds; oral tumors.
Axillary area: local injuries to hands, arms (e.g. lacerations, cat scratches, puncture wounds, etc.), skin lesions, breast lesions (tumor, abscess).
Femoral/inguinal node region: local injuries to feet, legs; skin lesions on feet, scrotal and perineal lesions.
Supraclavicular node region: history of smoking, pulmonary infection.

Associated Symptoms:
Pain; fever; chills; weight loss; skin rashes; discharges or change in appearance of lump (s).

Medical History:
Tuberculosis; infectious mononucleosis; recent sore throat; recurrent infections; venereal disease.

Medications:
Recent rubella or small pox vaccination; diphenylhydantoin (Dilantin).

Environmental History:
Exposure to measles, mumps, chickenpox; possible venereal disease exposure.

PHYSICAL EXAMINATION

Measure: temperature.
Skin: check lump for size, consistency, tenderness, fixation to adjacent tissues.
Nodes: If lump is probably not a lymph node: note pigmentation; note if smooth lump shows central dimpling on lateral pressure.
   If lump is probably a lymph node: check for other nodes; examine region drained by node; check for splenic enlargement.

GENERAL CONSIDERATIONS

Lymph nodes are palpable in the neck, under the jaw, around the ears, above the clavicle, under the arm, behind the knees and elbows, and in the inguinal regions. 'Lumps' located in these regions are usually lymph nodes.

This DIAGNOSTIC CONSIDERATIONS is organized into three basic categories:

1. Characteristics of lumps and lymphadenopathy.
2. Causes for lymphadenopathy.
3. Distinguishing characteristics of lumps that are not lymph nodes.

CHARACTERISTICS OF LUMPS AND LYMPH NODES

DIAGNOSTIC CONSIDERATIONS	HISTORY	PHYSICAL EXAM
Infection	Recent appearance (days); often tender.	Tender, warm and moveable mass; occasional purulent discharge and fever.
Malignancy	Slow change in size or appearance (weeks to months).	Infiltrating border; firm and often non tender and not moveable relative to adjacent tissues.
Benign growths	Long history or very slow change.	Often smooth nontender and freely moveable; numerous similar lesions may be noted.

CAUSES FOR LYMPH NODE ENLARGEMENT

1. <u>Generalized lymphadenopathy</u> is often associated with spleen enlargement.

COMMON DISEASE	FINDINGS
Viral disease (German measles, mumps, mononucleosis, chickenpox, toxoplasmosis).	Fever, skin rash may be present.

CAUSES FOR LYMPH NODE ENLARGEMENT

1. <u>Generalized lymphadenopathy</u> is often associated with spleen
   enlargement.

COMMON DISEASE	FINDINGS
Malignancy (lymphoma, leukemia)	Weight loss, fevers frequent; infections or bleeding tendency.
Other: Dilantin related.	Patient taking Dilantin.

2. <u>Localized lymphadenopathy</u> usually drains adjacent injury or
   infection.

LOCATION OF NODE	COMMON CAUSES
Cervical	Pharyngitis, dental caries, gingivitis, mononucleosis or German measles; rarely tuberculosis, tumor of head and neck, lymphoma.
Axillary	Arm infections; breast cancer; rarely lymphoma, cat scratch fever.
Femoral/inguinal	Foot, leg or groin infections; venereal diseases (syphilis, chancroid, lymphogranuloma inguinal); rarely lymphoma, melanoma or testicular cancer.
Supraclavicular	Usually cancer from lungs, abdomen or breast; rarely tuberculosis or lymphoma.

COMMON LUMPS	FINDINGS

   Smooth non-tender subcutaneous masses:

Lipoma	No change in size or appearance over years; soft; moves freely.

COMMON LUMPS   FINDINGS

Smooth non-tender subcutaneous masses:

Sebaceous cyst   Usually on face, scalp or
                                   trunk; may be noted to have
                                   periods of tenderness; may
                                   discharge white material;
                                   skin usually dimples on
                                   lateral pressure since
                                   the cyst is connected to
                                   the skin surface.

Smooth tender subcutaneous mass:

Abscess/pimple   Acute onset; tender and
                                   warm; may develop purulent
                                   drainage.

Raised, thickened, non-ulcerating lesions:

Warts   Children and young adults;
                                   most common on the fingers.

Seborrheic   Older patient; greasy or
keratosis   "crumbly" well demarcated
                                   brown lesions that appear
                                   stuck to the skin; usually
                                   on the trunk, face and
                                   extremities.

Keloids   History of trauma or in-
                                   flammatory lesion leading
                                   to over-exuberant scar
                                   formation. (Often family
                                   tendency for keloid
                                   reaction).

Raised thickened lesions that may ulcerate:

Basal cell   Older patient; slow growing;
carcinoma   pearly border; usually on sun-
                                   exposed areas; variable
                                   color; central necrosis
                                   may occur resulting in a
                                   flat chronic ulcer; rarely
                                   metastasize and cause local
                                   lymphadenopathy.

COMMON LUMPS   FINDINGS

Raised thickened lesions that may ulcerate:

    Squamous cell   Older patient; rapid growth;
    carcinoma   may produce large amounts
                                 of thickened horny material;
                                 may metastasize to local
                                 lymph nodes.

Pigmented lesions:

    Melanoma   Suggested by: variegated
                                 color (black, blue-gray,
                                 brown, pink); irregular
                                 border and irregular sur-
                                 face; later a change in
                                 size, darkening or ulcer-
                                 ation may occur; satellite
                                 lesions; itching or burn-
                                 ing sensation.

    Mole   Absence of above character-
                                 istics; usually uniform
                                 shades of brown.

    Seborrheic   See Raised lesions above.
    keratosis

    Hematoma   Acute onset usually follow-
                                 ing trauma; tenderness;
                                 blue discoloration (bruised).

Vascular lesions:

    Hemangiomas   Children: polyploid, raised
                                 bright red to purple; usually
                                 noted shortly after birth;
                                 often regress significantly
                                 by puberty.
                                 Adults: bright red raised
                                 small chronic lesions (so-
                                 called "cherry angiomas",
                                 common benign growths);
                                 rarely some large hemangiomas
                                 begin in later childhood and
                                 persist.

HISTORY

Descriptors:

General descriptors: refer to inside cover.

Associated Symptoms:

Oral growths; foul breath; sore or bleeding gums; recent
skin or genital lesions; "cold"; difficulty talking; difficulty swallowing; stridor; alcoholism; tooth ache; facial
pain; excessive or decreased salivation; fever; unpleasant
taste.

Medical History:

Diabetes; syphilis; alcoholism.

Medications:

Diphenylhydantoin (Dilantin); antibiotics; adrenal steroids.

Environmental:

Dentures; does patient smoke pipe, cigars or cigarettes; does
patient brush teeth regularly or use dental floss; recent
contact with a person with streptococcal pharyngitis.

PHYSICAL EXAMINATION

Measure: temperature.
Throat: (Do not use an instrument to examine the throat of a child
with drooling or stridor); check teeth, gums, pharynx for any
swelling, erythema, vesicles , petechiae or exudates.
Lymph nodes: check for cervical adenopathy.

DIAGNOSTIC CONSIDERATIONS	HISTORY	PHYSICAL EXAM
Primary gum disease:		
Gingival hyper-trophy	Patient is usually taking diphenylhydan-toin.	Gum hypertrophy.

DIAGNOSTIC CONSIDERATIONS	HISTORY	PHYSICAL EXAM
Primary gum disease: (Continued)		
Periodontal disease	Poor dental hygiene; sore bleeding gums.	Tooth plaque; hypertrophy of gingival papillae; gum recession with exposure of roots of teeth.
Primary lip disease:		
Herpes simplex	Painful lesions on lips or in mouth often recurring during viral infections.	Vesicles or round shallow ulcers.
Cheilosis	Chronic cracking and inflammation at the corners of the mouth; patients are often edentulous.	Angular fissures; marked inflammation occasionally present.
Growths and tumors of the mouth, lips and gums:		
Leukoplakia (premalignant lesion)	Patient is often a cigarette smoker; painless persistent white plaques.	White thickened patches not removeable with cotton swab.
Neoplasia	May note lumps or persistent sores; pain, gingival bleeding and unpleasant taste; cheek biting with cause benign "growths".	Firm, often ulcerated growth; swelling and redness of mouth with loose teeth and halitosis may be present.
Infections of the mouth, throat, lips and gums:		
Candida	Common in diabetics, infants and patients who have been on antibiotics or adrenal steroids; oral mucosa is sore; bleeding gums; unpleasant taste may be present.	White, creamy or curdy lesions with underlying red base.

DIAGNOSTIC CONSIDERATIONS	HISTORY	PHYSICAL EXAM

Infections of the mouth, throat, lips and gums:
(Continued)

"Trench mouth" (fusospirochetal infections)	Poor oral hygiene; halitosis.	Gingival bleeding; foul breath; gray membrane on pharynx.
Pharyngitis (streptococcal or viral)	Sore throat; recent contact with a person with streptococcal pharyngitis; may have associated malaise, earache, runny nose.	Fever; inflammed pharynx often with tonsillar swelling and exudate and enlarged tender anterior cervical lymph nodes.
Mononucleosis	Persistent sore throat ; lethargy.	Posterior cervical lymphadenopathy in addition to findings above.
Canker sore	Painful recurrent ulcers in the mouth or on the lips.	Vesicles and ulcers with erythematous edges; fever and lymphadenopathy are present occasionally.
Herpangina (usually pediatric)	Sudden sore throat; fever.	Fever; crops of vesicles and ulcers on the tonsils and soft palate; petechiae may be present.
Gingivostomatitis (Herpes simplex of children)	Fever and sore mouth.	Fever; vesicles and ulcers on tongue, gums and buccal mucosa; lymphadenopathy is common.
Peritonsillar abscess (usually pediatric)	Severe pain; difficulty talking and swallowing.	Fever; pharyngeal swelling that may push tonsil into pharnyx; lymphadenopathy.

DIAGNOSTIC CONSIDERATIONS	HISTORY	PHYSICAL EXAM

Infections of the mouth, throat, lips and gums: (Continued)

Epiglottitis (pediatric)	Children age 3-7; acute stridor; muffled speaking; sore throat; trouble swallowing; drooling.	Epiglottis enlargement may be present.

Oral manifestations of systemic disease:

Vitamin deficiency	Alcoholic patient and/or inadequate diet: sore tongue and mouth commonly occur in the malnourished patient.	Gingival bleeding; cheilosis of the angle of the mouth; oral ulcers; edematous, slick, fissured tongue with either atrophied or hypertrophied papillae.

Toothache:

Dental caries	At first only hurts with very hot or very cold food; eventually pain is constant; facial pain is common.	Tooth pain to direct palpation or percussion; anterior cervical lymphadenopathy or sinus tenderness occasionally present.
Sinusitis	Facial pain which often decreases when standing; nasal discharge.	Fever; sinus tenderness; nasal discharge may be present.

Drooling:

Normal	Children up to age 12 months; often worse when teething.	
Abnormal	Often associated with mental retardation, Parkinson's disease.	
Epiglottitis	See Infections of mouth, throat, lips and gums above.	

Reference: Harrison's Principles of Internal Medicine, Seventh Edition. Pages 199-204.

HISTORY

Descriptors:

General descriptors: refer to inside cover.
Is the weakness progressive, episodic or stable. When was
it first noted.
Location: generalized or localized weakness.
Aggravating factors: does the weakness become progressively
  worse with exercise or at the end of the day; is weakness
  most apparent when arising from a chair.

Associated Symptoms:
Neck or back pain; muscle pain or twitching; transient blurred
or double vision; changes in sensation or speech; heat intolerance, obesity or hirsutism.

Medical History:
Any chronic disease, particularly diabetes, alcoholism,
cervical or lumbar 'disc' disease; neurological disease;
thyroid disease.

Medications:
Adrenal steroids; diuretics.

Family History:
Muscle weakness; does it involve only men.

Environmental History:
Chronic insecticide exposure; past polio immunization.

PHYSICAL EXAMINATION

Neurological: Cranial nerves - note carefully if the facial
  muscles are normal and the extraocular movements are full.
  Strength and reflexes - is the weakness proximal or distal;
  are there fasciculations or muscle atrophy or tenderness.
  Sensation to pinprick or vibration; plantar reflex.

GENERAL CONSIDERATIONS

The complaint of muscle weakness must be distinguished
from a weak feeling when no actual weakness exists (see
LETHARGY) or the sudden onset of muscle weakness usually
associated with a cerebrovascular accident (see STROKE).

DIAGNOSTIC CONSIDERATIONS	HISTORY	PHYSICAL EXAM
Myopathy		
Dystrophy	Progressive bilateral proximal muscle weakness; difficulty arising from a chair; often a family history affecting male children.	Proximal muscle wasting except in the childhood type where muscles may appear "big" but weak (particularly 'pseudohypertrophy of calves'); Reflexes present but decreased.
Myositis	Proximal muscle weakness and pain.	Proximal muscle wasting and tenderness.
Secondary Myopathies		
disuse atrophy	Often a history of chronic muscle disuse (following cerebrovascular accidents, rheumatoid arthritis); weakness may be localized.	Atrophy and contractures in unused muscles. Reflexes are usually present but variable in intensity.
drug related	Alcohol, steroids and diuretics (low potassium); weakness is usually generalized.	Diffuse weakness often more marked in proximal muscles.
endocrine disease (hyperthyroidism or adrenalism)	Heat intolerance may be noted in hyperthyroidism and truncal obesity or hirsutism noted in hyperadrenalism. Weakness is usually generalized.	Diffuse weakness often more marked in proximal muscles. Atrophy may be present.

DIAGNOSTIC CONSIDERATIONS	HISTORY	PHYSICAL EXAM

Neuromuscular Disease

(Myasthenia or insecticide poisoning) — Easy fatigueability; generalized weakness; diplopia and weakness of speech are common; weakness is worse at the end of the day. — Decreased strength with any repetitive exercise often returning to normal after rest; reflexes decrease with progressive tapping.

Neuropathy

(Diabetes; alcoholism; spinal disc pressure; direct nerve injury or ischemia) — Change in sensation is often noted; weakness is often localized. — Distal weakness with atrophy and occasional fasciculations; sensation often decreased. Reflexes are weak or absent.

Weakness secondary to localized lesions in the spinal cord or brain (demylinating disease; tumor; cerebrovascular accident; tumor; cervical spondylitis). — Localized weakness and abnormal sensation are frequently noted. — Localized muscle weakness often with hyperreflexia and a Babinski response. Sensation is often abnormal.

Special Considerations:

Guillian Barré Syndrome or Tick bite paralysis — Symmetric weakness and paralysis beginning in legs. May be rapidly progressive. — Flaccid symmetric paralysis; decreased reflexes. Abnormal sensation and cranial nerve abnormalities are frequently present. (A tick will be found in the scalp if tick bite paralysis).

DIAGNOSTIC CONSIDERATIONS	HISTORY	PHYSICAL EXAM

Special Considerations:

Poliomyelitis	Fever, and rapid onset of widespread weakness. No history of previous polio immunization.	Fever initially; asymetric flaccid paralysis; reflexes are often decreased and the cranial nerve examination is usually abnormal.
Amyotrophic Lateral Sclerosis (adult) or Werdnig and Hoffman disease (pediatric).	Slowly progressive often asymmetrical weakness in the adult or diffuse weakness in the child.	Muscle weakness and atrophy with fasciculations and normal sensory examination. Reflex changes are variable in the adult. Reflexes are usually absent in the child.

HISTORY

Descriptors:

General descriptors: refer to inside cover.

It is often more revealing to examine the nails before obtaining any history.

Aggravating factors: trauma, constant water immersion or chemical contact, nail biting.

Associated Symptoms:
Pain; swelling or redness; discoloration, pitting or nail destruction; any adjacent skin lesions; scaling skin lesions on elbows or knees.

Medical History:
Chronic lung disease; chronic heart disease; thyroid disease; diabetes, psoriasis.

Family History:
Similar nail problems.

Environmental History:
Chemical contacts or frequent water immersion.

PHYSICAL EXAMINATION

Extremities: check for clubbing of fingers, nail pitting or destruction; inflammation of surrounding tissue.

DIAGNOSTIC CONSIDERATIONS	HISTORY	PHYSICAL EXAM
Nail Pain		
Hematoma	Usually follows direct trauma.	Blue black discoloration under the nail.
Glomus tumor	Severe recurrent pain, often following minimal trauma.	Small pink growth under the nail.

NAIL PROBLEMS
(Continued)

DIAGNOSTIC CONSIDERATIONS	HISTORY	PHYSICAL EXAM
Nail Bed Inflammation		
Bacterial, yeast infection.	Often follows constant immersion or trauma to nails; seems to be more common in diabetic patients.	Redness, swelling of surrounding skin; eventually nail destruction.
Nail Destruction		
Fungus infection.	May follow constant immersion.	Nail destruction with little tissue reaction.
Psoriasis	History of scaly skin lesions on extensor surfaces of extremities; past diagnosis of psoriasis.	Pitting of nails with eventual nail destruction; little tissue reaction.
Nail Biting	History of nail biting habit.	Nail destruction.
Common Nail Changes of Generalized Disease		
Clubbing	History of chronic lung or heart disease is often noted; may be familial. Rarely associated with carcinoma or chronic infections.	Bulbous deformity of the finger tip with rounding of the nail where it meets the nail bed.
Separation of Nails From Nail Beds	Usually traumatic or secondary to occupation; rarely associated with thyroid disease.	Partial or complete separation of nail from nail bed.

DIAGNOSTIC CONSIDERATIONS	HISTORY	PHYSICAL EXAM
Nail Growth		
Warts	Painless growths most often in adolescents.	Gray brown or flesh colored "vegetative" appearing lesions.
Other (carcinoma, melanoma, gradually enlarging masses, cysts).	Usually asymptomatic.	Are not wartlike in appearance.

HISTORY

Descriptors:

General descriptors: refer to inside cover.
Character: what if anything has been thrown up; how much.
Aggravating factors: possibility of pregnancy; recent
  contaminated food, alcohol ingestion; motion sickness;
  recent cessation of adrenal steroid medication.

Associated Symptoms:
Fever; vertigo; ear ringing; headache or change in motor
function or mental function; excessive thirst; chest pain;
diarrhea or abdominal pain; black bowel movements or
vomiting blood; light stools, dark urine or jaundice;
muscle aches.

Medical History:
Diabetes; peptic ulcer disease; cardiovascular disease;
pregnancy.

Medications:
Any.

Environmental History:
Recent contact with others suffering from nausea and vomiting,
or hepatitis.

PHYSICAL EXAMINATION

Measure: blood pressure, standing and lying; temperature;
  pulse.
Eyes: check carefully for nystagmus; fundi: absent   venous
  pulsations, papilledema.
Throat: odor of ketones on breath.
Abdomen: tenderness; distention or abnormal tympany; bowel
  sounds.
Rectal: check stool for occult blood.
Special: if possible, check vomitus for occult blood.

DIAGNOSTIC CONSIDERATIONS	HISTORY	PHYSICAL EXAM
Acute gastroenteritis (See DIARRHEA for further consideration)	Nausea and vomiting frequently accompanied by diarrhea, muscle aches and mild fever; may occasionally follow contaminated food injestion.	Mild fever; minimal if any abdominal tenderness to palpation.
Acute Hepatitis	History similar to gastroenteritis above. Light stools, dark urine or jaundice may be noted. Contact with others who have had hepatitis.	Liver tenderness or enlargement is often present.
Abdominal emergency (See ABDOMINAL PAIN for further considerations)	Abdominal pain; high fever; vomiting blood; melena; history of ulcer occasionally.	Postural drop in blood pressure or persistent abdominal tenderness may be present. Stool may be positive for occult blood; bowel sounds may be absent.
Following ingestion of medications, chemicals or alcohol.	Many medications or chemicals cause nausea and vomiting.	Usually normal.
Early pregnancy	Last menstrual period more than 6 weeks ago.	Often unremarkable.
Labyrinthine disorders (See DIZZINESS (vertigo)).	Vertigo; ear ringing; motion sickness.	Nystagmus may be present.

DIAGNOSTIC CONSIDERATIONS	HISTORY	PHYSICAL EXAM
Chronic "indigestion"	Chronic nausea without vomiting.	Normal.

Relatively uncommon causes of nausea and vomiting:

Diabetic acidosis	History of diabetes; loss of appetite; polyuria; excessive thirst.	Eventually progresses to rapid pulse, postural drop in blood pressure, slow mental function and ketones on breath; bowel sounds may be absent.
Adrenal insufficiency	Often follows sudden withdrawal of adrenal steroids; abdominal pain; irritability.	Postural drop in blood pressure; lethargy; occasional fever.
Brain swelling	Headache; changes in mental or motor function.	Elevated blood pressure and slow pulse, papilledema and absent retinal vein pulsations may be present.
Myocardial infarction	Chest pain; sweating; history of cardio-vascular disease.	Often normal. Blood pressure may be low and pulse irregular.

Reference: Harrison's Principles of Internal Medicine. Seventh Edition. Pages 211 - 213.

HISTORY

Descriptors:

General descriptors: refer to inside cover.
Onset: when first noted.
Character: type and amount of vomiting; how frequent.
Aggravating factors: fright; excitement; certain foods
  (specify); possibility of drug or poison ingestion.
Relieving factors: burping the infant.

Associated Symptoms:
Fever; weight loss; headache; ear ache; sore throat; vomiting
blood; abdominal distention; diarrhea; decrease in bowel
movements; crying on urination; dark urine.

Medications:
Any.

Environmental History:
Recent contact with others suffering from vomiting, hepatitis.

PHYSICAL EXAMINATION

Measure: pulse, weight, height. Compare to growth chart.
Eyes: Fundi - absent venous pulsations, or papilledema.
Neck: stiffness.
Abdomen: check for distention, masses, apparent tender-
  ness.
Rectal: stool for occult blood.
Skin: turgor; purpura.
Special: if possible, check vomitus for occult blood.

GENERAL CONSIDERATIONS

Abdominal Pain - See ABDOMINAL PAIN - PEDIATRIC.

Abdominal Trauma - See TRAUMA.

DIAGNOSTIC CONSIDERATIONS	HISTORY	PHYSICAL EXAM
Acute Gastro-enteritis or Systemic Infection (see DIARRHEA-ACUTE PEDIATRIC for other considerations)	Acute vomiting and fever often accompanying many childhood infections (e.g. otitis media, tonsillitis, kidney infection). Diarrhea may be noted.	Fever is common. Normal abdominal examination. Abnormal ear or throat exam may be present.
Hepatitis	As in acute gastroenteritis above. Dark urine and a contact with someone who has had hepatitis may be noted.	Hepatic tenderness or enlargement.

Gastrointestinal Obstruction

High bowel obstruction (pyloric stenosis or duodenal atresia)	Persistent vomiting with large amounts of food in vomitus. No bile in vomitus. May vomit blood. Usually noted in first 3 months of life.	Weight loss. Decreased skin turgor may be noted as well as a flaccid abdomen by examination.
Lower bowel obstruction (intussusception, Hirschprung's disease, meconium plug)	Green bile in vomitus. Abdominal distention. Decrease or cessation of bowel movement. Rare in the child over 2 years of age.	Abdominal distention and hyperresonance. Absent bowel sounds alternating with high pitched rushes. Stools may be positive for occult blood.
Normal Infantile Regurgitation	Variable amount and frequency of vomiting. Often related to excessive stimulation after feeding. May be relieved by burping the infant frequently.	Normal examination.

DIAGNOSTIC CONSIDERATIONS	HISTORY	PHYSICAL EXAM
Cerebral Irritation (meningitis, brain tumor)	Head holding, headache, lethargy or projectile vomiting may be noted. Symptoms progress over hours to days.	Fever, decreased pulse, and stiff neck are common. Bulging fontanels or papilledema may be noted.
Following Poison or Medication Ingestion	History of ingestion may be noted.	May be normal.
Resulting from "Metabolic Disease" (gluten sensitivity phenylketonuria)	Newborns may begin vomiting soon after birth or later in life as certain foods are introduced.	Weight loss, and decreased skin turgor may be present.
Unclear (functional)	The older child may vomit from fright, excitement or to get attention.	Normal.

HISTORY

Descriptors:

    General descriptors: refer to inside cover.
    Onset: trauma; car accident.
    Aggravating factors: raising arms over head; hyperex-
      tension of neck.

Associated Symptoms:
    Headache; any change in strength or sensation; fever of
    chills; swelling or tenderness of neck; shoulder pain;
    chest pain; nausea or vomiting.

Medical History:
    Cardiovascular disease; any neurological disease; rheuma-
    toid or degenerative arthritis; malignancy.

Medications:
    Phenothiazines.

PHYSICAL EXAMINATION

    Measure: temperature.
    Neck: range of motion; tenderness.
    Neurological: reflexes; strength and sensation in upper and
      lower extremities.
    Special: observe if downward pressure on the head while the
      patient has his neck hyperextended, turned to the right and
      turned to the left reproduces or exacerbates the pain.

DIAGNOSTIC CONSIDERATIONS	HISTORY	PHYSICAL EXAM
Referred pain to the neck.	Anterior neck pain in the adult suffering from intrathoracic disease, particularly angina or myocardial infarction.	Normal neck exam.
Pain of Muscle strain	Dull ache over back of neck; a recent history of injury or strain (typical whiplash injury in car accident) is often obtained.	Neck muscle spasm or tenderness.

DIAGNOSTIC CONSIDERATIONS	HISTORY	PHYSICAL EXAM
Pain of Cervical disc disease or arthritis	Occipital headache; numbness or shooting pain in shoulders, arms or hands; rarely weakness in arms or legs may be noted.	Decreased range of motion of neck; cervical compression test may produce pain; abnormal neurological examination is occasionally present.
Neck Pain from infection or tumor infiltration of cervical vertebra	Persistent posterior neck pain; sometimes severe.	Direct tenderness of the spinal process to pressure and percussion; rarely changes in muscle strength and reflexes are present.
Neck Pain from meningismus	Aching, stiff neck; headache; fever; nausea and vomiting may be noted.	Fever and neck rigidity on attempted flexion is frequently present.
Dystonic reaction	Painful involuntary spasm of neck, muscles or jaw. Patient may have recently begun to take phenothiazine medications.	Spasms of the neck musculature are apparent.
Painful Neck Lumps	See LUMP - LYMPHADENOPATHY.	
Neck Trauma	See HEAD TRAUMA or TRAUMA.	

Reference: Harrison's Principles of Internal Medicine. Seventh Edition. Pages 42 - 43.

HISTORY

Descriptors:

    General descriptors: refer to inside cover.
    Onset: are complaints noted only during certain seasons of
      the year.
    Location: does the problem involve one or both nostrils.
    Aggravating factors: trauma; nose picking; possible foreign
      body; does contact with any substances cause the symptoms.
    Past treatment or evaluation: sinus x-rays; nasal examination;
      nasal packing, cautery or surgery in past.

Associated Symptoms:

    Fever or chills; swollen glands; facial or sinus pain; upper
    respiratory infection; bruising or bleeding tendency; change
    in smell; eyelid swelling or visual disturbances.

Medical History:

    Diabetes; hypertension; bleeding disorder; asthma; nasal
    polyps; allergies (specify); neurological disease.

Medications:

    Warfarin (Coumadin); nasal sprays (decongestants); anti-
    biotics.

Environmental History:

    Is there a possibility of foreign body in the nose.

PHYSICAL EXAMINATION

    Measure: temperature; blood pressure.
    Head: Sinus exam - sinus tenderness.
    Nose: check for growths, bleeding points, septal deviation
      and inflamed mucosa.
    Neck: cervical nodes: enlargement; tenderness.

DIAGNOSTIC CONSIDERATIONS	HISTORY	PHYSICAL EXAM
Epistaxis (Bloody nose)	Anterior bleeding due to nose picking or occasionally in association with chronic nasal-sinus infection. Posterior nose bleeding occasionally	Fresh blood in the pharynx usually indicates a posterior nasal bleed; hypertension is occasionally present. Anterior septal spurs,

DIAGNOSTIC CONSIDERATIONS	HISTORY	PHYSICAL EXAM
Epistaxis (Bloody nose)	occurs with severe chronic disease (blood disorders, hypertension). Anticoagulants can worsen bleeding problem.	signs of nasal trauma or excessive mucosal dryness may be present with anterior bleeding.
Runny, stuffy nose	Acute runny, stuffy nose is due to viral upper respiratory infection; a chronic runny stuffy nose is usually a manifestation of excessive decongestant use, or allergies. Chronic allergic rhinitis (or sinusitis) often is worse during different seasons of the year.	Pale, boggy nasal mucosa, clear discharge and nasal polyps may be present.

Purulent nasal drainage:

Acute sinusitis	Sinus tenderness; facial pain; rarely visual disturbances or swollen eyelids if sphenoid or ethmoid sinus infection. Pain relieved by standing.	Fever; sinus tenderness. Purulent sinus-nasal discharge.
Chronic sinusitis	Persistent purulent discharge or mild sinus aches are often the only manifestations; diabetes predisposes to severe infections.	Often normal. Purulent drainage may be present in the nose.

DIAGNOSTIC CONSIDERATIONS	HISTORY	PHYSICAL EXAM
Purulent nasal drainage:		
Persistent unilateral sinus drainage		Occasionally septal deviation, tumors or foreign bodies are present in the nose.
<u>Nasal Polyps</u>	Often a history of asthma.	Polyp.
<u>Changes in smell</u>	Actual loss of smell or alterations of smell may be noted following infection, trauma; rarely noted in neurological disease.	Purulent nasal discharge may be present.

HISTORY

Descriptors:

General descriptors: refer to inside cover.
Onset: is the numbness chronic, acute or transient.
Location: where is the numbness noted; is it unilateral or
  bilateral.
Aggravating factors: relation to trauma or cold; recent
  prolonged pressure on area or sites proximal to numb
  area.

Associated Symptoms:

Headache; anxiety/depression; numbness in hands or around
mouth; weakness; muscle wasting or tenderness; incoordination; change in vision, speech or hearing; neck pain;
back pain.

Medical History:

Any neurological disease; cardiovascular disease; diabetes;
high blood pressure; emotional problems; alcoholism;
anemia; syphilis; tumor; kidney disease.

Medications:

Isoniazid; Nitrofurantoin (Furadantin).

Environmental History:

Arsenic; lead.

PHYSICAL EXAMINATION

Measure: blood pressure, pulse.
Pulses: check pulses in any numb extremities; if patient is
  over 40: check strength of carotid pulses and listen for
  bruit.
Neurological: carefully outline the numb areas using sensa-
  tion to pinprick and vibration to "map out" the deficit.
  Check muscle strength,deep tendon reflexes and plantar reflex.
  Have patient walk heel to toe; perform finger to nose test.

GENERAL CONSIDERATIONS

Numbness is the awareness of the loss of cutaneous sensation, but in common usage patients often preferentially use
the term "numbness" to describe pins and needle sensation
(paresthesia) or dull pain. The most common causes for numbness, tingling or pain in the extremities are discussed under

GENERAL CONSIDERATIONS

JOINT-EXTREMITY PAIN, FOOT-ANKLE PAIN, HAND-WRIST-ARM PRO-
BLEMS. Other causes are summarized below.

DIAGNOSTIC CONSIDERATIONS	HISTORY	PHYSICAL EXAM
Acute reversible numbness:		
Hyperven-tilation	Bilateral hand "numb-ness"; faintness; paresthesia around lips; dyspnea.	Normal physical exam; hyperventila-tion may reproduce symptoms.
Transient ischemic attack	Usually unilateral numbness coupled with clumsiness and at times trouble speaking and see-ing; old age; cardiovascular disease, hypertension, or dia-betes are predis-posing factors.	Carotid bruits may be heard; physical exam often normal between attacks.
Demyli-nating disease	Often multiple epi-sodes involving different areas and eventually leaving residual deficit.	Neurological abnormal-ities may be present transiently. With recurrent attacks multiple of neuro-logical changes be-come apparent.
Nerve compres-sion	See below.	See below.

DIAGNOSTIC CONSIDERATIONS	HISTORY	PHYSICAL EXAM

Chronic often irreversible numbness:

Peripheral neuropathy (often in alcoholism, diabetes, chronic renal disease, pernicious anemia, drug related (isoniazid) or toxic metals (lead or arsenic)	Numbness and weakness often noted in a fixed distribution.	Glove and stocking, distal and often symmetrical sensory loss to pinprick and vibration are present. Decreased reflexes and strength in involved areas may also be present.
Central nervous system damage (tumor, cerebrovascular disease, syphilis)	Changes in sensation, strength and co-ordination are often noted.	Abnormal reflexes, and decreased sensation are present. Decreased ability to define objects and decreased strength may also be present.
Nerve Compression	Usually a unilateral complaint of sharp pains or numbness in an extremity. Often secondary to direct pressure on a nerve (particularly at the axilla, elbow, knee, or wrist); concurrent back or neck pain may be noted.	Decreased sensation and reflexes may be present in the distribution of the affected nerve.

Reference: Harrison's Principles of Internal Medicine. Seventh Edition. Pages 110 - 116.

HISTORY

Descriptors:

General descriptors: refer to inside cover.
Onset: at what age was the patient first obese; what is his
lowest and highest weight after attaining adult height.
Aggravating factors: usual number of meals per day; does
the patient eat between meals; what emotional stresses
lead to excessive eating; motivation for weight loss.
Past treatment or evaluation: results of past dieting.

Associated Symptoms:

Edema; cold intolerance; easy bruising; change in skin or
hair texture; depression or anxiety.

Medical History:

Cardiovascular disease; diabetes; thyroid disease; hypertension; gout; emotional problems.

Medications:

Diuretics; digitalis; reserpine; diet pills (specify).

Family History:

Obesity.

Environmental History:

Other people's attitudes toward problem and diet; family
and work problems.

PHYSICAL EXAMINATION

Measure: blood pressure; weight.
General: body habitus and distribution of fat.
Extremities: edema.
Skin: striae; plethora; edema; hair and skin texture.
Neurological: Reflexes - carefully observe relaxation phase.

GENERAL CONSIDERATIONS

The obese person eats more calories than his level of
activity requires. Overeating is usually the result of
cultural and emotional habits. The frequency of food ingestion is an important determinant of fat synthesis; the
fewer the meals, the more calories are converted to fat from
each meal. Obese people have a tendency to develop gout,
diabetes, hypertension and cardiovascular disease.

GENERAL CONSIDERATIONS

Very few obese patients suffer from endocrine disorders. The patient with Cushing's disease often complains of weakness and has striae of the skin, excessive fat over the back of the neck, and fat distributed on the trunk rather than the extremities. Hypothyroid patients are not usually grossly obese. They may have cold intolerance, deepening of the voice and thickening of the hair and skin. The relaxation phase of deep tendon reflexes is often prolonged.

Reference: Harrison's Principles of Internal Medicine. Seventh Edition. Pages 232 - 236.

HISTORY

Descriptors:

General descriptors: refer to inside cover.
What was ingested; how much; when.
Aggravating factors: had the patient been contemplating
  suicide; what is the age and weight of patient.

Associated Symptoms:

Loss of consciousness; hyperactivity; abnormal breathing;
fever or low temperature; change in skin color; convulsions,
tremors or spasms.

Medical History:

Previous overdose, poisoning, or suicide attempts; depression; emotional problems; alcohol or drug abuse; any chronic
disease.

Medications:

What medications were available to the patient.

PHYSICAL EXAMINATION

Measure: blood pressure; pulse; respiratory pattern and
  rate; temperature.
Mental Status: is the patient oriented to his surroundings,
  the time and the date; is the patient stuporous or coma-
  tose.
Throat: staining of oral mucosa; odor of breath.
Chest: rales, rhonchi or wheezes.
Skin: needle tracts; jaundice; cyanosis; cherry red color.
Neurological: pupil size and reactivity to light; response
  to pain; deep tendon reflexes.

GENERAL CONSIDERATIONS

The best treatment of poisoning is prevention of accidental
ingestion by keeping all medications and chemicals out of
the reach of children. In adults prevention is best directed
at recognizing the person who is prone to suicide (See SUICIDE).

The first task of the examiner is to assure that the patient's
vital signs are stable. Supportive measures for respiratory
depression and hypotension should be begun at once. The next
goal is to ascertain as accurately as possible the name of the

GENERAL CONSIDERATIONS

suspected poison, the amount ingested and the interval
between probable ingestion and discovery. The age and
weight of the patient should also be determined. All
suspected toxic substances and their containers should
be examined and retained for possible further evaluation.

Nonspecific treatment of poisoning may be begun before
the identity of the drug or chemical is known. The most
commonly available treatment regimens involve either in-
duction of emesis (15-20 ml syrup of ipecac followed by
2 glasses of water) or gastric lavage to prevent further
absorption of poison. However, this form of treatment is
contraindicated when strong corrosives (acids/alkali) have
been ingested more than 30 minutes prior to evaluation.
Liquid hydrocarbons which may damage the lungs should only
be removed after a cuffed endotracheal tube has been inserted to prevent aspiration of gastric contents. An endotracheal tube should also be passed with the comatose or
convulsing patient before gastric lavage or emesis is
undertaken. Children often spill substances which they
have ingested; children ingesting corrosives, hydrocarbons
or pesticides should be thoroughly bathed.

Specific treatment of poisoning may involve the use of
antidotes, cathartics, diuretics, administration of agents
which enhance excretion, exchange transfusions, chemical
neutralization of the poison, and dialysis. Specific
treatment depends on the knowledge of the identity and
action of the poison. Ingestion of more than one poison
at a time is common.

Information regarding specific treatment can be readily
obtained from:

1. Harrison's Principles of Internal Medicine. Seventh
   Edition. Pages 649 - 695.
2. M. W. Gleason, Clinical Toxicology of Commercial Pro-
   ducts, Williams and Wilkins, Baltimore, 1969.
3. Local poison control centers.
4. Regional poison control centers and their telephone
   numbers:
   Athens, Georgia: 404-549-9977.
   Chicago: 312-942-5000.
   Denver: 303-758-0403.
   Kansas City: 816-421-8060.
   Los Angeles: 213-664-2121.
   Memphis: 901-522-3000.
   New Orleans: 504-899-3409.
   New York: 212-340-4495.
   San Francisco: 415-431-2800.

HISTORY

Descriptors:

General descriptors: refer to inside cover.
Onset: how long do the attacks last; have there been previous attacks.
Aggravating factors: relation to exercise, emotion, standing.
Past treatment or evaluation: was the pulse rate taken during spell; how fast was it; were the beats regular or irregular; was onset and cessation gradual or abrupt.

Associated Symptoms:
Anxiety; depression; giddiness; weakness; tingling in hands or around mouth; fever; chills; chest pain; trouble breathing.

Medical History:
Cardiovascular disease; diabetes; high blood pressure; thyroid disease; blood disease; emotional problems; alcohol.

Medications:
Antidepressants; digitalis or other heart pills; bronchodilators or decongestants (e.g. Sudafed); thyroid.

Environmental History:
Cigarette smoker; alcohol; tea; coffee.

PHYSICAL EXAMINATION

Measure: temperature; blood pressure and pulse standing and lying.
Neck: thyroid enlargement.
Chest: lungs for rales.
Heart: gallops or murmurs.

GENERAL CONSIDERATIONS

Chest pounding, "flipping of the heart" and heart fluttering are frequently noted when a person is tense or anxious. Missed beats are infrequent and the heart rate and rhythm are normal. Anxiety induced palpitations do not usually signify cardiac dysfunction.

DIAGNOSTIC CONSIDERATIONS	HISTORY	PHYSICAL EXAM
Anxiety/ depression	Normal heart rate; often symptoms of hyperventilation (tingling in hands and around mouth); the depressed patient is frequently concerned about heart function.	Normal.
Drug related	Palpitations may be related to taking coffee, tea, bronchodilators, antidepressants, digitalis, thyroid.	Extrasystoles or tachyarrhythmias (usually more than 120 beats per minute) are often noted.
Primary cardiac dysfunction	Often a history of angina, myocardial infarction or congestive heart failure.	Extrasystoles, tachyarrhythmias (more than 120 beats per minute) irregularly irregular rhythm, gallops and murmurs may be noticed.

Associated with other disease:

		Usually manifested by a fast regular resting heart rate and:
Fever	Fever; chills.	Temperature elevation.
Anemia and/ or postural hypotension	Faintness or palpitation particularly on minimal exertion or sudden standing.	Pallor and/or postural hypotension.
Thyroid disease	Heat intolerance and weight loss.	Usually palpable thyroid. Tremor may also be noted.

Reference: Harrison's Principles of Internal Medicine.
Seventh Edition. Pages 182 - 184.

PIGMENT CHANGE
(i.e. too dark or too light; if <u>red</u> see SKIN PROBLEMS)

HISTORY

Descriptors:

General descriptors: refer to inside cover.
Onset: when noted.
Location: generalized or localized.
Aggravating factors: relation to sun, clothing; pregnancy.

Associated Symptoms:
Weight loss; hair loss; pain, itching of lesion.

Medical History:
Adrenal disease; liver disease; thyroid disease.

Medications:
Phenothiazines (Stelazine, Thorazine); anti-malarials;
nicotinic acid; birth control pill.

Family History:
Similar problems.

Environmental History:
Constant trauma to involved area; chemical/rubber contact.

PHYSICAL EXAMINATION

Measure: blood pressure.
Skin: carefully examine and note if problem is diffuse or
circumscribed; are there blisters or signs of irritation.

DIAGNOSTIC CONSIDERATIONS	HISTORY	PHYSICAL EXAM
Generalized increase of pigmentation:		
Adrenal insufficiency	Weight loss; nausea; diarrhea.	Hypotension; diffuse tan skin with accentuation in skin creases.
Porphyria Cutanea Tarda	Family history; sun exposed areas.	Tan skin and or blisters in exposed areas.

DIAGNOSTIC CONSIDERATIONS	HISTORY	PHYSICAL EXAM
Generalized increase of pigmentation:		
Jaundice	See JAUNDICE	Icteric sclera.
Drug	See above drugs.	Often skin darkening.
Localized increase of pigmentation:		
Pregnancy or taking birth control pill. (cloasma, melasma)	History of pregnancy or taking birth control pill.	Malar area often involved; nipples darker.
Tinea Versicolor	See below.	
Generalized decrease of pigmentation:		
Albino	Similarly afflicted blood relatives.	Light blue iris; blond/white hair.
Localized decrease of pigmentation:		
Vitiligo	Occasionally a history of endocrine disease.	Well demarcated and complete pigment loss.
Secondary to trauma	Often a history of repeated trauma, scratching, or chemical contact (particularly rubber).	Often thickened and/or irritated skin.
Tinea Versicolor	White or tan flat areas usually over the trunk. Some scaling is common.	White or tan scattered or confluent patches or plaques.

Reference: Harrison's Principles of Internal Medicine. Seventh Edition. Pages 273 - 281.

HISTORY

Descriptors:

General descriptors: refer to inside cover.
Onset: when was the last menstrual period; was pregnancy
  desired; precise age of patient.
Aggravating factors: history of German measles or skin rash
  with "swollen glands" in first trimester; previous miscarriages; previous children of low birth weight; premature, very large or jaundiced babies; pregnancy in last
  12 months; previous multiple pregnancies; I.U.D. possibly
  still in place.
Past treatment or evaluation: has the patient been examined
  for this pregnancy. What were the results of this examination.

Associated Symptoms:

Breast enlargement; nausea and vomiting; vaginal discharge
or spotting; fetal "kicking"; fever or chills; burning or
frequent urination; ankle swelling.

Medical History:

Diabetes; hypertension or previous toxemia of pregnancy;
sickle cell disease; heart disease or rheumatic fever; drug
addiction; previous uterine or pelvic surgery (particularly
ceasarian delivery); known single kidney or kidney disease.

Medications:

Any. Particularly fertility drugs.

Family History:

Any familial diseases; mongolism.

Environmental History:

Marital status; family-job security; financial status; number of children and their ages.

PHYSICAL EXAMINATION

Measure: blood pressure, weight.
Abdomen: fundus height; what is the fetal heart rate and
  where is it best heard.
Pelvic exam: check carefully for the presence of adnexal
  swelling or a short cervix. Pelvic examination is
  generally not performed in the third trimester.
Extremities: varicosities or edema.

GENERAL CONSIDERATIONS

Pregnant females generally note nausea, vomiting, breast enlargement and vaginal discharge or mild spotting in the first trimester. Fetal movement is normally noticed at the 16th week at which time abdominal enlargement is usually apparent.

A primary consideration in the first prenatal visit is the identification of the high risk pregnancy that will require special treatment to insure the health of the mother and child.

The pregnancy is at high risk if:
1. the mother is less than 18 or over 35.
2. the mother has any of the "aggravating factors", personal or familial history of diseases listed in the medical history above.
3. the mother is obese, hypertensive or has an abnormal pelvic examination particularly as listed above.
4. the pregnancy is unwanted or the home and personal circumstances of the mother are inadequate.

HISTORY

Descriptors:

General descriptors: refer to inside cover.
Onset: at what age did (does) the child seem retarded. How
was this 'retardation' first manifested.
Aggravating factors: is apparent retardation worsened when
the child is required to use his vision or hearing. Is
the child worse when emotionally upset.
Past treatment or evaluation: previous well baby, eye, hearing and reading examinations; results of these evaluations.

Associated Symptoms:
Abnormal hearing, vision, emotional behavior; convulsions;
motor or sensory disturbances.

Medical History:
Mother: during pregnancy: rash and lymph node enlargement,
german measles, unusually long or short labor, prolonged
anesthesia, toxemia of pregnancy.
Child: prematurity; convulsions at birth; deformities;
low APGAR score; jaundice.

Family History:
Retardation; deafness; familial disease; Jewish background.

Environmental History:
Possibility of lead, paint or dirt eating; frequent family
moves or school changes; apparent family disharmony.

PHYSICAL EXAMINATION

Measure: developmental milestones (see WELL BABY CHECK);
head circumference; height and weight.
Ears: check for ability to turn to noise or recognize
whispered sounds. Check ears for obstruction, perforated
drums.
Eyes: be sure child follows objects; do a visual acuity.
screen (when possible). Check fundus for cherry red
spots or degeneration.
Abdomen: check for liver or spleen enlargement.

GENERAL CONSIDERATIONS:

The diagnosis of retardation

There is wide variation in the rate of development expe-

GENERAL CONSIDERATIONS

The diagnosis of retardation

rienced by normal children. Between two and four months it
is easy to underinterpret development. Assessment becomes
more accurate at six to seven months when more milestones
are present to evaluate.

Before the diagnosis of mental retardation is considered,
several serial developmental examinations performed at bi-
monthly intervals should show that the child is subnormal in
several areas of development. Most children so followed will
show that they are "slow starters" who achieve normal development. The diagnosis of retardation should never be made
except by persons comfortable with developmental neurology
because of social impact of the diagnosis.

Marked discrepancies in different areas of development should
be considered due to environmental influences (child neglect,
frequent school changes) or diseases affecting specific areas
of the body (muscle disease, poor vision, poor hearing, lead
toxicity or neurological disease).

Children born of mothers who had rubella in the first trimester or toxemia during any stage of pregnancy have an increased risk of being mentally retarded at a later time.
Children born with jaundice, seizures, a low APGAR score,
"cerebral palsy", mongolism or prematurity also have an increased risk of mental retardation. Infantile hypothyroidism, a rare but easily treatable disorder, will invariably
cause retardation if not recognized at an early age. Clues
to the diagnosis of hypothyroidism include increasing
weight relative to height, yellow skin, thick tongue and
slow development.

HISTORY

Descriptors:

General descriptors: refer to inside cover.
Onset: is problem chronic or of relatively recent onset.
Male: decreased interest; failure of erection; failure
  of ejaculation; premature ejaculation.
Female: decreased interest; pain on intercourse; failure
  of orgasm.

Associated Symptoms:

Genital lesions; vaginal or penile discharge; genital
pain; back pain; calf or buttock pain caused by exercise
and relieved by rest; anxiety; depression; change in
sleep pattern, appetite; change in bowel or bladder function; spontaneous erections.

Medical History:

Cardiovascular disease; diabetes; hypertension; venereal
disease; infertility or sterility; recent surgery; neurological disease; emotional problems; past history of
being sexually assaulted (rape).

Medications:

Guanethidine (Ismelin) or methyl-dopa (Aldomet).

Environmental History:

Family or job problems; is patient being told to seek help
on insistence of the sexual partner.

PHYSICAL EXAMINATION

Genital: check distribution of pubic hair. Is it normal
  for the sex of the patient. Check perineal sensation
  to pinprick.
Female: Pelvic exam. Check for genital lesions, atrophy
  of the vaginal mucosa, pelvic tenderness, vaginal stenosis, clitoral adhesions.
Male: Size on consistancy of testicles. Reflex contraction of anus to squeezing of glans penis.
Pulses: femoral and pedal pulses.

GENERAL CONSIDERATIONS

Emotional problems are the commonest cause of sexual dysfunction. Frequently, sexual problems are a sign of trouble

GENERAL CONSIDERATIONS

in the relationship between partners. Males often note that they can have spontaneous erections but seem to be unable to sustain it under "appropriate" circumstances. Females often are unable to attain orgasm and may complain of discomfort during sexual intercourse although physical examination is normal.

Genital abnormalities in the female may cause pain on intercourse or lack of adequate sensation. The atrophic vagina of the post-menopausal female and post childbirth trauma are considered common causes of genital discomfort. The male taking guanethidine or methyl-dopa, with claudication, or if diabetic with autonomic neuropathy may be unable to sustain erection or attain ejaculation.

Neurological causes for sexual problems are relatively uncommon. Spontaneous erections do not occur. They are usually associated with bowel or bladder dysfunction and decreased perineal sensation or loss of the bulbocavernosus reflex in the male.

Hormonal causes for sexual dysfunction are rare; they are usually associated with abnormal pubic hair distribution and abnormal secondary sexual characteristics.

Finally, chronic diseases of any type may interfere with sexual interest or function.

Reference: Harrison's Principles of Internal Medicine.
Seventh Edition. Pages 248 - 249.

HISTORY

Descriptors:

General descriptors: refer to inside cover.
Onset: how old was the child when illnesses began; describe previous illnesses; when and how were previous illnesses documented; how old is the child now.
Aggravating factors: do illnesses usually follow emotional upsets.

Associated Symptoms:

Is child small for age; recurrent wheezing attacks; cough; sputum production; frequent bulky stools; exercise intolerance; crying or complaint of burning on urination.

Medical History:

Recurrent pneumonias; meningitis; bone, skin, ear or sinus infections; cystic fibrosis; asthma.

Medications:

Any.

Environmental History:

Home environment (cleanliness, heat, running water, dust and pets); description of family; are brothers and sisters of school age.

False Positive Considerations:

See discussion below.

PHYSICAL EXAMINATION

Measure: weight, height, head circumference (if less than 2 years of age).
Ears: perforation, opacity or poor movement of ear drum to pneumo-otoscopic pressure. Check hearing.
Chest: check lungs for any abnormalities.
Heart: check for murmurs.
Abdomen: check for masses.
Extremities: check for finger clubbing, cyanosis or edema.

GENERAL CONSIDERATIONS

The anxious or inexperienced parent may worry that a child is

GENERAL CONSIDERATIONS

sick frequently because the parent is unaware that even the "average" child may have five to ten illnesses each year. Furthermore, the child born into a family where the siblings are of school age may seem to get more communicable diseases than older brothers and sisters who are exposed to communicable diseases at school and transmit them to the younger sibling. Allergic rhinitis or asthma may cause a child to be 'sick' frequently. A history of wheezing is usually obtained. Occasionally the older attention-seeking child may offer frequent complaints, but this behavior which the parent would not easily recognize as being "emotional", is probably uncommon. Growth is generally normal in all the circumstances listed above.

The child with recurrent, documented infections other than "colds" may be suffering from severe underlying disease (cystic fibrosis, immune deficiency or asthma); this child often does not grow and develop as expected. Further evaluation is indicated.

HISTORY

Descriptors:

General descriptors: refer to inside cover.
IT IS OFTEN HELPFUL TO EXAMINE THE LESION BEFORE OBTAINING
ANY HISTORY. THE NATURE OF THE LESION MAY BE APPARENT.
Onset: how did the problem start; is it healing or spreading.
Location: one lesion or several lesions; major locations or
regions of involvement.
Character: itching; scaling; crusting; weeping; blistering.
Describe lesions as they initially appear and their evo-
lution.
Aggravating factors: scratching; skin contact with obvious
irritant (poison ivy, wool, etc.).
Past treatment or evaluation: has a previous diagnosis been
given; skin biopsies done in past; treatment with antihistamines, adrenal steroid pills or creams. Effects of
these attempted remedies.

Associated Symptoms:
Fever; chills.

Medical History:
Diabetes; kidney disease; asthma; hay fever; skin diseases
(eczema, psoriasis, contact dermatitis).

Environmental History: •
Contact with persons with a similar problem; nature of work;
exposures to dusts, chemicals and pets.

PHYSICAL EXAMINATION

Measure: temperature.
Skin: note the color, location, and other characteristics of
the skin lesions (see below).

GENERAL CONSIDERATIONS

Description of dermatological lesions is the key to accurate
diagnosis. Primary lesions (the first lesions which usually
appear) are:
Flat (macule) - color change only.
Raised solid lesions - nodule if more than 1 cm, papule
if less .
Blister - vesicle if less than 1 cm, bulla if larger .

<u>GENERAL CONSIDERATIONS</u>

> Pus pocket (pustule) - elevated lesion filled with purulent material.
> Cyst - a lesion with an internal wall that contains blood or fluid .

Secondary lesions occur because of the natural evolution of the primary lesion or because of scratching. The common secondary lesions are:
> Scaling.
> Crusting - dried blood cells, serum.
> Scratches (excoriation).
> Erosions - superficial focal loss of skin.
> Ulcers - focal loss of skin and underlying tissue. Healing leads to scars.
> Fissures - linear losses of skin and underlying tissues .
> Scars.

Other common but relatively unique skin lesions are:
> Thickening of the epidermis (lichenification)
> Petechiae - Specks of blood in skin which do not blanch when pressed.
> Telengiectasias - Dilation of superficial vessels.
> Deposits of blood in skin larger than 1 cm (Purpura).
> Hives (urticaria).

Skin changes may indicate serious underlying disease. <u>Purpuric skin lesions</u> should be carefully managed since they are frequently associated with severe infections (eg. systemic spread of meningococcus infection, gonorrhea or Rocky Mountain spotted fever). <u>Pruitus</u> alone, without obvious evidence of skin disease, is usually due to dry skin, but occasionally biliary cirrhosis, kidney disease or cancer may present in this fashion. Finally, reactions to medications may occur at any time after ingestion and the '<u>drug rash</u>' may show characteristics of most of the primary or secondary skin responses listed above.

The commonest skin problem in all age groups is <u>eczematous dermatitis</u>. Redness, vesicles, papules, crust and scales may be noted at various stages of development. It may follow direct contact with certain substances (poison ivy, medications, cosmetics, etc.), be a response to sunlight (often combined with a medication), or be due to poor circulation in the legs (stasis dermatitis). Eczematous dermatitis may also be a skin reaction to ill defined environmental agents conditioned by genetically determined factors (atopic eczema,

<u>GENERAL CONSIDERATIONS</u>

    neurodermatitis, lichen simplex). Secondary bacterial
infection of eczematous dermatitis is an occasional problem.

    Other common adult and pediatric considerations are listed
below. The list is not complete and is provided only as a
brief survey of common non-eczematous skin diseases.

DIAGNOSTIC CONSIDERATIONS	FINDINGS

<u>Chronic</u>:

    Warts, moles, other chronic papules and nodules: see LUMP-
LYMPHADENOPATHY.

Acne (adolescent)	Blackheads, whiteheads, pustules and inflammatory papules over face, and often the back, chest and shoulders.
Fungus infections:	
Scalp	Scaling red plaques with hair loss and broken hairs.
Body	Itching, scaling inflamed plaques consisting of confluent vesicles and papules; eventual central healing with peripheral spread of the lesion (so called 'ring worm').
Groin	Marginated symetrical itching, red scaling lesions with advancing actively inflamed borders.
Feet and hands	Itching; vesicles on the palms and soles; scaling and fissuring between toes.
Psoriasis (adult)	Well circumscribed silvery scaled plaques on scalp, knees and elbows; may involve nails, groin or entire trunk; removal of scale may reveal small bleeding points; itching is common.

DIAGNOSTIC CONSIDERATIONS	FINDINGS

Chronic

Seborrheic Derma-
titis

Poorly demarcated greasy scaled plaques on scalp, eyebrows and nasolabial areas; may involve back of ears, chest and groin.

Acute/recurrent:

Bacterial infections

Impetigo (pediatric)

Red papules and superficial vesicles which become confluent producing the characteristic honey colored crust. The lesions often heal centrally while spreading. Most often located on head and neck and diaper area of in-fants   impetigo is also contagious and may appear anywhere.

Boils

Tender superficial abscesses that usually occur in the hair bearing areas.

Hives (urticaria)

Itching; migratory pink itchy wheals (skin swelling); often follows drug, shellfish or unusual food ingestion; rarely throat involvement may com-promise breathing.

Infestations:

Scabies

Itching bites (papules and vesicles) characteristically in warm moist body folds, between fingers, at the nipples, navel, knees and groin; Examination often reveals burrows (zig-zag thread-like channels) with variable degrees of inflammation. Scabies is contagious.

Lice (head, body
or pubic types)

Itching; papules; urticaria and even-tual secondary bloody crusts confined to hair bearing areas. Nits can be seen on the hairs. Lice are contagious.

DIAGNOSTIC CONSIDERATIONS	FINDINGS

Acute/recurrent:

Pityriasis Rosacea
(young adults)

Oval salmon colored superficially scaling plaques along trunk; preceded by a large initial patch that remains throughout the illness (herald patch). This eruption is self limited.

Tinea Versicolor

Flat, barely palpable superficial scaling plaques over neck, shoulder and trunk; may look tan on light skin or light on dark skin.

Yeast infections
(Candida)

Red moist grouped papules and pustules. More common in diabetics and children; itching or pain is common. More often located in areas of skin exposed to chronic moisture (groin, base of nails).

Common Pediatric Rashes

Chicken Pox

Umbilicated vesicles principally on the trunk which crust within several days of onset; successive crops of vesicles appear in the next 2-5 days.

German Measles

Fever; posterior cervical node enlargement for up to 7 days followed by sudden red finely papular 'blushing' rash on face which fades after one day and is followed on the second day by the same rash on the trunk and extremities.

Measles

Cough; fever; conjunctivitis for 3 days followed by generalized purple red macular and papular rash starting at head and spreading over body in 3 days. Throat examination often reveals characteristic red spots with small white centers (Koplik's spots).

Reference: Harrison's Principles of Internal Medicine.
            Seventh Edition. Pages 252 - 260.

HISTORY

Descriptors: refer to inside cover.
How long has the baby been thought to be small; what was the baby's birth weight and height; what has been the pattern of it's growth; any recent change in growth; has mother weighed baby pre- and post-breast feeding.

Associated Symptoms:
Cough; breathing trouble; exercise intolerance; cyanosis; anorexia; foul greasy bowel movements; vomiting; constipation; diarrhea (note the frequency and amount); fever; behavior problems; lethargy.

Medical History:
Any chronic disease; past serious illnesses now "cured".

Medications:
Any.

Family History:
Small stature; cystic fibrosis; renal disease.

Environmental History:
Stability of family; recent stresses (births, deaths, hospitalizations); dietary history.

PHYSICAL EXAMINATION

Measure: weight; height; head circumference; temperature; pulse; blood pressure.
Throat: presence of tonsillar tissue.
Chest: rales, wheezes.
Heart: murmurs.
Abdomen: masses.
Extremities: muscle firmness and tone.
Skin: rashes, infection.
Nodes: any enlargement.
Neurological: reflexes.

GENERAL CONSIDERATIONS

Most "small babies" are constitutionally small, often reflecting the size of other family members. Inadequate diet is the next most common cause of "small babies".

GENERAL CONSIDERATIONS

Discrepancies in height, weight and head circumference are suggestive of underlying disease. If these discrepancies are not diminished after several successive examinations further evaluation for more serious disease is indicated.

DIAGNOSTIC CONSIDERATIONS	HISTORY	PHYSICAL EXAM
Inadequate feeding of child	Usually associated with poor education of the mother in child care; occasionally part of the "battered child" syndrome; rarely parents may fear "overfeeding" the child; (in the tropics, insufficient fluid may be provided to the child with normal meals.)	Weight often increases less than height (height is closer to normal than weight); an actual weight loss may occur; eventually buttocks become wasted and abdomen protruberant.
Fibrocystic disease	Frequent respiratory infections; family history of fibrocystic disease; foul, greasy stools.	Weight often increases less than height (height is closer to normal than weight); an actual weight loss may occur; eventually buttocks become wasted and abdomen protruberant.
Enzyme deficiency diseases	Diarrhea, greasy bowel movements and occasional vomiting usually follows ingestion of milk or other foods.	Weight often increases less than height (height is closer to normal than weight); an actual weight loss may occur; eventually buttocks become wasted and abdomen protruberant.
Hypothyroidism	Prolonged jaundice at birth; constipation; mottled skin as newborn.	Continued weight gain with premature plateau of length; umbilical hernia, slow

DIAGNOSTIC CONSIDERATIONS	HISTORY	PHYSICAL EXAM
		relaxation phase of reflexes and decreased muscle tone may be noted.
Other chronic disease and infections: Chronic lung disease, renal disease, cardiac disease, intestinal parasites.	History of chronic disease.	Weight often increases less than height (height is closer to normal than weight); an actual weight loss may occur; eventually buttocks become wasted and abdomen protruberant; fever; abnormalities of heart, lungs or abdomen may be noted.
"Growth Lags"	During and immediately after illness or other severe stresses the child's growth may have ceased or decreased and never completely "returned to normal."	Physical exam usually normal except for low height and weight of the child.

HISTORY

Descriptors:

General descriptors: refer to inside cover.
Past treatment or evaluation: how does patient know of the
  diagnosis of gallstones; gallbladder xray done in past.

Associated Symptoms:
Pain in the right upper quadrant or upper back; nausea; vomiting; jaundice; dark urine; light stools; fever; chills;
food intolerance (specify).

Medical History:
Anemia; liver disease or jaundice; obesity;
abdominal surgery; pancreatitis.

Family History:
Gallstones; anemia.

PHYSICAL EXAMINATION

Measure: temperature.
Eyes: scleral icterus.
Abdomen: masses or tenderness in right upper quadrant.

GENERAL CONSIDERATIONS

See ABDOMINAL PAIN.

Reference: Harrison's Principles of Internal Medicine.   Seventh
             Edition.   Pages 1561 - 1565.

HISTORY

Descriptors:

General Descriptors: refer to inside cover.
  Blurred vision only -- see EYE PROBLEMS or DOUBLE VISION.
  Loss of speech -- see TALKING TROUBLE.
  Numbness only noted -- see NUMBNESS.

Onset: was functional deficit maximal at onset or did it
  develop gradually or stepwise. Was the problem solely
  motor or were there several kinds of deficits. Precisely
  describe the type of neurological functions affected and
  the order in which the deficits appeared.

Aggravating factor: position of body at time of problem.

Past treatment or evaluation: previous skull x-rays, lumbar
  punctures, cerebral arteriograms.

Associated Symptoms:

Headache; stiff neck; fever or chills; nausea/vomiting;
blurred vision; disequilibrium; trouble speaking or swallowing; motor or sensory change; seizures; loss of consciousness.

Medical History:

Diabetes; cardiovascular disease; hypertension.

Family History:

Diabetes; cardiovascular disease; hypertension.

Medications:

Warfarin (Coumadin); antiarrhythmic drugs, birth control
pills; antihypertensive medications.

PHYSICAL EXAMINATION

Measure: blood pressure; pulse lying and standing; respirations; temperature.

Eyes: fundus exam for hemorrhages, exudates, papilledema;
  check for absence of venous pulsations.

Pulses: carotid pulses -- listen carefully for bruit; palpate
  for differences in strength.

Heart: murmurs; gallops; rhythm.

PHYSICAL EXAMINATION
  (Continued)

    Neurological, complete: check for differences in strength,
      sensativity, coordination and reflexes between sides; care-
      fully elicit the plantar reflex.

GENERAL CONSIDERATIONS

    The major question is whether or not the patient is, in fact,
    having a "stroke". This requires that the examiner be able
    to recognize the common "stroke" syndromes.

    For therapeutic convenience, cerebrovascular occlusive disease
    is arbitrarily divided into three categories:

    1. The transient ischemic attack (TIA): a reversible episode
       of neurological deficit lasting no longer than 24 hours.

    2. Stroke in evolution: patients may note that the neurologi-
       cal deficit progresses in a stepwise fashion over hours to
       days until it culminates in a completed "stroke".

    3. Completed stroke: a fixed neurological deficit of several
       days duration.

       TIA and "stroke in evolution" syndromes often precede
       developement of cerebral infarction.
       Thus recognition and appropriate treatment of the early
       signs of imminent cerebral infarction may potentially save
       the patient from permanent brain damage.

    Hemorrhagic cerebrovascular accidents, on the other hand,
    usually present few warning symptoms. They are characterized
    by sudden severe headache, nausea, vomiting, rapid develop-
    ment of neurological deficits and loss of consciousness.
    Papilledema and a stiff neck are frequently present.

GENERAL CONSIDERATIONS
(Continued)

The pattern of the TIA, stroke in evolution or the completed
stroke is often a clue to the anatomic location of the brain
dysfunction.

Vertebrobasilar artery occlusive disease often presents with:
vertigo; bilateral blurring, loss of vision or double vision;
syncope; bilateral, unilateral or occasionally alternating
motor or sensory deficits.

Carotid artery occlusive disease is characterized by:
hemimotor, hemisensory and hemivisual deficits with associated
speech abnormalities if the dominant hemisphere is involved.
Transient contralateral monocular blindness may also occur
(amaurosis fugax).

Reference: Harrison's Principles of Internal Medicine. Seventh
             Edition. Pages 1743 - 1780.

HISTORY

Descriptors:

General descriptors: refer to inside cover.
What precisely does the patient plan to do; does he only
have a vague notion of killing himself or has he made specific plans; why; marital status of patient.

Associated Symptoms:
Anxiety; depression; peculiar thoughts; feeling of losing control of his mind; feelings of persecution.

Medical History:
Emotional problems; previous suicide attempts; alcoholism;
drug abuse; any physical illness.

Medications:
Any.

Family History:
Suicide.

Environmental History:
Losses (financial, death, separation from loved ones); does the
patient have someone at home who can provide emotional support.

PHYSICAL EXAMINATION

Mental Status: orientation, memory, ability to calculate;
bizarre thoughts; delusions.

GENERAL CONSIDERATIONS

Suicidal thoughts occur commonly. Over one half of those
who commit suicide give a warning. Therefore, it is important to identify those persons expressing suicidal thoughts
who are at high risk to attempt suicide.
The risk of suicide is greater in the presence of any of the
following: Alcoholism; physical illness; a family history of
suicide; history of previous attempts; specific plans for
"how to" commit suicide; recent loss or a single, divorced or
widowed marital status; psychosis.

Reference: Harrison's Principles of Internal Medicine. Seventh
Edition. Pages 1894 - 1895.

HISTORY

Descriptors:

General descriptors: refer to inside cover.
Location: exactly where is it noted; is it generalized or
localized to an extremity or the abdomen.
Aggravating factors: menses; position; trauma; drugs; certain foods or dust; time of day; type of feeding (pediatric);
pregnancy.
Past treatment or evaluation: results of most recent EKG
or chest X-ray; renal and liver function tests.

Associated Symptoms:
Weight change; shortness of breath; jaundice; itching;
tenderness, redness or aching of the involved area; chronic
loose stools; abdominal pain.

Medical History:
Cardiovascular disease; kidney disease; varicose veins;
anemia; bowel disease; liver disease; allergies; past trauma
or surgery in or near involved area.

Medications:
Diuretics (Lasix, Diuril); digitalis; adrenal steroids; birth
control pills.

Family History:
Edema; swelling.

Environmental History:
Poor nutrition.

PHYSICAL EXAMINATION

Measure: blood pressure (standing, lying); pulse; weight.
Neck: veins for distention at 90^0.
Chest: rales.
Heart: cardiac enlargement; murmurs; gallops.
Abdomen: distention; shifting dullness; fluid wave; hepato-
splenomegaly or other masses; resonance to percussion (pedi-
atric).
Extremities: are there varicose veins in the involved area;
is the edema pitting or non-pitting; are there any skin
changes (redness, warmth, discoloration).

DIAGNOSTIC CONSIDERATIONS	HISTORY	PHYSICAL EXAM
Systemic Disease		
Cardiac, renal or liver failure	History of these diseases; Dyspnea and orthopnea may be noted.	Pitting edema; cardiac gallops or murmurs, rales and ascites are often noted; facial edema may be most prominent in children with nephrotic syndrome.
Toxemia of pregnancy	Often asymptomatic initially.	Pitting edema; hypertension; enlarged uterus.
Hypoalbuminemia (malnutrition or excessive kidney or bowel loss of protein)	History of weight loss, poor dietary intake or chronic diarrhea.	Pitting edema; wasted buttocks and protruberant abdomen usually present; hair coarsening and depigmentation may occur.
Anemia (high output failure)	Often asymptomatic; may complain of shortness of breath.	Pitting edema; pallor; resting tachycardia.
Angioedema	Sudden swelling that may cause severe shortness of breath or abdominal pain. Often is a familial problem and may follow minimal trauma, infection or exposure to specific foods or dusts.	Non-pitting edema; patient may develop respiratory stridor; in children the edema may be primarily facial.
Nonspecific swelling (cyclic edema of women)	"Bloating," weight gain, or mild swelling often associated with menses or birth control pills; often cyclical variation in weight during the day.	Minimal pitting edema. Otherwise normal examination.

DIAGNOSTIC CONSIDERATIONS	HISTORY	PHYSICAL EXAM
Local Disease		
Lymphatic blockage	Adults may notice a-symptomic swelling of extremities without previous history of varicose veins or thrombophlebitis. Occasionally secondary to filariasis, tumor invasion, surgery or radiation of involved area.	"Woody" or rubbery non-pitting edema.
Venous disease (thrombophlebitis and venous insufficiency)	Often starts during or after attacks of painful swelling in the legs; the patient complains of chronic aching; night cramps and itching are common.	<u>Acutely</u>: warmth, tenderness, redness and pitting edema. If in calf, dorsiflexion of foot may cause increased pain (Homan's sign). <u>Chronically</u>: brown purple discoloration; skin thickening and non-pitting woody edema.
Infection (cellulitis) (usually pediatric)	Often facial swelling after infection of tooth, sinus or skin.	Warmth, redness and tenderness of skin. Localized swelling, usually asymetric.
Abdominal "Swelling"		
Ascites	Often a history of liver disease; less frequently history of cancer, heart or renal disease.	Shifting dullness, fluid wave, splenomegaly often present; extremities often wasted; pitting leg edema often noted.
Obesity	Usually asymptomatic.	Normal exam except for generalized obesity.
Pediatric causes	Any of above. Masses (bladder, tumor, etc.).	As above. Mass felt.

SWELLING
(Continued)

DIAGNOSTIC CONSIDERATIONS	HISTORY	PHYSICAL EXAM
Pediatric causes	Air swallowing after feeding (infants).	Hyperresonant abdomen after feeding, otherwise normal.
	Normal toddler habitus.	Normal child.

Reference: Harrison's Principles of Internal Medicine. Seventh Edition. Pages 176-182.

HISTORY

Descriptors:

General descriptors: refer to inside cover.
Onset: is problem stuttering, use of nonsense words, total inability to speak; is the patient right-handed or left-handed.
Pediatric: at what ages were vocalization, words, intelligible speech, sentence usage, good sentence structure first noted.

Associated Symptoms:

Headache; seizures; numbness or weakness anywhere; change in vision; trouble hearing; change in swallowing; anxiety.

Medical History:

Stroke; high blood pressure; cardiovascular disease; diabetes; neurological disease; emotional problems.

Medications:

Anticoagulants.

Family History:

Speech disorders.

Environmental History:

Change in job, family, school; birth injury.

PHYSICAL EXAMINATION

Ears: can patient hear watch tick; perform Rinne and Weber tests; check for obstruction of the ear canal or perforation of the ear drum.
Neck, adult: check both carotid pulses for differences in strength of pulse and bruit.
Neurological: deep tendon reflexes; can patient see, name objects, read and repeat names.

TALKING TROUBLE
(Continued)

GENERAL CONSIDERATIONS

Acquired speech abnormalities in the adult are often caused by cerebrovascular disease and the patient often seeks medical attention because of other associated neurological deficits in addition to the speech problem (see STROKE).

Children frequently suffer from problems of articulation, particularly between ages 3 and 5 when "stammering", "stuttering" and mispronunciation of sounds is common. Generally. a normal 4 year old, except for occasional problems with articulation, uses completely intelligible sentences.

Mental retardation, hearing dysfunction, emotional stress and developmental abnormalities of the central nervous system, palate and lip may all contribute to persistent "talking troubles" of the child.

An acute change in the child's voice associated with drooling and a sore throat may be due to epiglottitis (see HOARSNESS).

Reference: Harrison's Principles of Internal Medicine. Seventh Edition. Pages 137-148.

HISTORY

Descriptors:

General descriptors: refer to inside cover.
  Describe symptoms specifically.
Aggravating factors: history of trauma.
Relieving factors: does lying flat reduce pain or swelling.

Associated Symptoms:

Undescended or hypermobile testicle; testicular pain, swelling or
masses; fever; chills; nausea; dysuria, blood in urine; scrotal
skin lesions; swollen lymph nodes.

Medical History:

Hernia; mumps; kidney stones.

PHYSICAL EXAMINATION

Measure: temperature.
Rectal: prostate examination. If child and no testicles are
  felt, check carefully for the presence of a uterus.
Genital: inguinal canal; check for an inguinal hernia. Check
  for testicular or scrotal mass. If a mass is present is it
  tender or hard - can it be transilluminated. Examine children in Buddha position.

DIAGNOSTIC CONSIDERATIONS	HISTORY	PHYSICAL EXAM
Testicular Pain		
Infection (Epididymitis)	Testicular pain, dys-uria, tenderness and swelling; onset usually over hours. May be secondary to mumps (orchitis).	Rectal exam may reveal prostate tenderness. Fever and a tender swollen testicle usually noted.
Tortion of the testicle	Patient usually 5 to 20 years old. Sudden onset of severe pain, nausea.	The testicle is usually tender and swollen.
Pain referred to the scrotum.	The pain of renal colic is often referred to the testicle; flank pain is usually present	Normal exam.

DIAGNOSTIC CONSIDERATIONS	HISTORY	PHYSICAL EXAM
Pain referred to the scrotum.	and gross blood in the urine is noted in a third of the patients.	
<u>Testicular Mass</u>	Patient usually notices the mass. Usually painless.	
Hydrocoele	Occasionally enlarges when crying (pediatric)	Turgid mass, transilluminates.
Spermatocele		Soft mass separate from the testicle.
Varicocele	Vague scrotal discomfort decreased by lying flat. Painless mass.	Soft mass that feels like a "bag of worms" which may collapse when patient lies down.
Tumor	Painless mass.	Firm, fixed mass on testes.
Hernia	Often a large mass that may "fall back" into the abdomen.	Herniated bowel easily separated from testicle. Does not transilluminate; bowel sounds may be heard over the scrotum.
<u>Other</u>		
Absent or undescended testicles in children.	Usually testicles descend by one year of age. Occasionally mobile testis descend intermittently.	Testes may be noted to draw into inguinal canal. If not present in Buddha position check carefully for abnormalities of the penis and the presence of a uterus on rectal examination.

HISTORY

Descriptors:

General descriptors: refer to inside cover.
Past treatment or evaluation: results of previous thyroid tests.

Associated Symptoms:

Prominent eyes; heat or cold intolerance; change in skin or
hair texture and distribution; voice change; anxiety/depression;
neck mass or pain; change in bowel or menstrual patterns;
change in weight, appetite.

Medical History:

Cardiovascular disease; eye disease; hyper or hypothyroidism;
goiter; thyroid surgery or radioactive treatment of thyroid.

Medications:

Thyroid hormone (Cytomel, thyroid extract, Synthroid); anti-
thyroid agents - propylthiouracil (PTU); methimazole, (Tapa-
zole).

Family History:

Thyroid disease or goiter.

False Positive Considerations:

"Thyroid" trouble is often used freely to describe obesity
or anxiety; "goiter" could be any other neck swelling.

PHYSICAL EXAMINATION

General: does patient appear nervous and hyperactive or
hypoactive.
Measure: blood pressure; resting pulse; temperature; weight.
Eyes: lid lag; exophthalmos; extraocular movements.
Neck: thyroid: size, firmness, nodules.
Extremities: tremor; sweating.
Skin: fine or coarse hair.
Neurological: ankle jerk - slow or abnormally fast relaxa-
tion phase.

GENERAL CONSIDERATIONS

Patients with undiagnosed thyroid disease usually present
with one of a variety of common symptoms (anxiety, depression,
palpitations, menstrual irregularities, weight loss, tremor,

GENERAL CONSIDERATIONS

heat or cold intolerance, changes in bowel habits). While
thyroid disease is not often the cause of these complaints,
it must always be considered in such patients because appropriate treatment usually leads to dramatic improvement.

DIAGNOSTIC CONSIDERATIONS	HISTORY	PHYSICAL EXAM
Hyperthyroidism	Nervousness; irritabil-lity; weight loss; heat intolerance; increased prominence of eyes; de-creased menstrual flow.	Tachycardia; lid lag; exophthalmos; enlarged thyroid; warm, moist skin; tremor; abnormally fast relaxation of ankle jerk; weight loss may be marked.
Hypothyroidism (may follow therapy for hyperthyroidism)	Cold intolerance; deep-ened voice; excessive menstrual flow; consti-pation.	Thick, dry, coarse skin; coarse hair; slow re-laxation phase of deep tendon reflexes; en-larged firm thyroid and a hoarse "froggy" voice may be noted.
Thyroid Pain (thyroiditis)	Anterior neck or jaw ache lasting several weeks.	Enlarged tender thryoid.
Thyroid Enlarge-ment. ("goiter")	Usually asymptomatic. Chronic enlargement is rarely associated with hyper or hypo-thyroidism. Pro-gressive enlargement over weeks or months is suggestive of thy-roid cancer.	Diffusely enlarged thy-roid. Stoney hard en-largement is suggestive of cancer. Signs of hy-per and hypothyroidism listed above are occa-sionally noted.
Thyroid Nodule	Usually asymptomatic. progressive enlarge-ment over weeks or months is suggestive of thyroid cancer.	Thyroid nodule.

Reference: Harrison's Principles of Internal Medicine. Seventh
            Edition. Pages 465-484.

HISTORY:

Descriptors:

General Descriptors: refer to inside cover.
    When, where and how did the injury occur.
Past treatment or evaluation: last tetanus injection.

Medical history: any chronic disease.

Medications: any.

Environmental: did injury occur at work.

PHYSICAL EXAMINATION:

Measure: blood pressure; pulse: respiratory rate and pattern.
Special: stop any bleeding by applying direct pressure or
    tourniquet. Establish an airway if necessary. Elevate the
    legs and prepare for intravenous therapy if systolic blood
    pressure is less than 90 mm of mercury.

GENERAL CONSIDERATIONS:

The primary consideration in trauma is first to recognize
whether the patient is in immediate need of life support
or has a high probability of requiring life support or surgical intervention. Thus, maintenance of an adequate airway
and control of bleeding and shock are priorities. There-
after those persons who have received severe head trauma,
gunshot wounds, stab wounds or blunt trauma to the chest
and abdomen must be carefully evaluated and regularly
observed for possible decompensation of vital signs and
shock.

Further considerations for specific locations of trauma are
listed on the following pages.

HEAD TRAUMA:
(See also HEAD TRAUMA)

HISTORY:
Unconsciousness; amnesia for pre-injury events; vomiting
following injury; localized weakness; sensory loss or
incoordination.

PHYSICAL EXAM:
Mental status: orientation to time, place, person.
Head and neck: check head and neck for discoloration,
  laceration, point tenderness, bony malalignment of
  the skull.
Ears: check tympanic membranes for discoloration.
Nose: check for clear discharge.
Neurological: cranial nerve function; deep tendon reflexes;
  sensation to pinprick; strength of extremities; plantar
  response.

DIAGNOSTIC CONSIDERATIONS	HISTORY	PHYSICAL EXAM
Neck fracture	Neck pain	Neck tenderness; malalignment of neck or paralysis of extremities may also be noted.
Skull fracture	Unconsciousness more than 5 minutes; loss of memory for event preceding injury; complaints of nonvisual neurological abnormalities following the trauma.	Abnormal mental status; bony malalignment of the skull; ear drum discoloration; bilateral black eyes; localized neurological abnormalities.

CHEST TRAUMA

HISTORY:
Breathing trouble; vomiting or coughing up blood after injury.

PHYSICAL EXAMINATION:
Measure: blood pressure checking for pulsus paradoxicus.
Neck: check height of jugular venous pulse; check for tracheal deviation.
Chest: check for rib tenderness; observe chest for adequate symmetric movement on inspiration; percuss and listen to the lungs noting any differences between sides.
Heart: listen for clarity of heart sounds.

DIAGNOSTIC CONSIDERATIONS	HISTORY	PHYSICAL EXAM
Pneumothorax	Dyspnea; chest pain.	Chest wall tenderness; unilateral increased resonance to percussion and decreased breath sounds; trachea may be deviated.
Hemothorax	Dyspnea; chest pain.	Chest wall tenderness; unilateral decreased resonance to percussion and decreased breath sounds; tracheal deviation may be noted.
Cardiac Tamponade	Dyspnea.	Disappearance of pulse with inspiration or pulsus paradoxicus, more than 10 mm of mercury; diminished heart sounds; elevation of jugular venous pulse.
Flail chest	Dyspnea; chest pain.	Multiple rib fractures and inward movement of the chest on inspiration is obvious.
Injury of lung tissue	Dyspnea; coughing up blood.	Chest wall tenderness.

CHEST TRAUMA
(Continued)

DIAGNOSTIC CONSIDERATIONS	HISTORY	PHYSICAL EXAM
Airway obstruction	Dyspnea.	Decreased breath sounds; exaggerated inspiratory effort with little air movement.

ABDOMINAL TRAUMA

HISTORY:
Abdominal pain; blood in urine.

PHYSICAL EXAMINATION:
Measure: blood pressure and pulse standing and lying.
Abdomen: check for abdominal tenderness, mass or rigidity.
 Note if bowel sounds are present. Check for puncture wound
 of abdomen or abdominal bruises. Check pelvis for stability.
Rectal exam: check for tenderness. Examine stool for occult
 blood.

DIAGNOSTIC CONSIDERATIONS	HISTORY	PHYSICAL EXAM
Laceration of internal organs or occult bleeding	Abdominal pain; blood in urine may be noted.	Postural drop in blood pressure may signify blood loss; a penetrating wound may be noted; probablity of severe injury is increased if the patient has abdominal tenderness, rigidity; decreased bowel sounds or bruising of the abdominal skin.

PELVIC PAIN

HISTORY:
Blood in urine; inability to void; numbness or decreased strength in lower extremities.

PHYSICAL EXAMINATION:
Measure: blood pressure and pulse standing and lying.
Abdomen: check for pelvic displacement or increased mobility of the pubic or iliac bones. Look for perineal bruising.
Extremities: look for leg length discrepancy.
Neurological: check reflexes and sensation in lower extremities.

DIAGNOSTIC CONSIDERATIONS	HISTORY	PHYSICAL EXAM
Pelvic fracture (often associated with severe internal bleeding)	Pain on weight bearing or direct pelvic pressure; changes in strength and sensation in legs may rarely be noted; blood in urine is frequently noted.	Postural drop in blood pressure may signify blood loss; bruising of perineum; displacement of pelvic bones; increased mobility of pelvic bones; neurological abnormalities may be noted.
Urethral tear	Blood in urine or decreased ability to void.	Usually the same findings as pelvic fracture above.

EXTREMITY TRAUMA

PHYSICAL EXAMINATION:
Extremity: check pulses, skin temperature, ability to move and sensation of limb distal to injury; check joints for mobility, stability and swelling; check for displacement, tenderness or swelling of any bones.

<u>EXTREMITY TRAUMA</u>
(Continued)

   <u>PHYSICAL EXAMINATION</u>:
   (Continued)

   <u>Special</u>: Remove any materials that might become impossible
      to remove if the injured area swells.

DIAGNOSTIC CONSIDERATIONS	HISTORY	PHYSICAL EXAM
Nerve or vessel injury	Insensitivity or loss of ability to move the injured extremity.	Pallor; coldness or decreased pulses distal to injury; decreased sensation or muscle weakness distal to injury may be noted.
Fracture or dislocation	Inability of the injured area to function normally is usually noted.	Displacement deformity or unusual mobility of the involved area; tenderness and swelling are frequently noted.
Open fracture		Bone protrudes through wound or skin.

<u>NECK OR BACK TRAUMA</u>

   <u>HISTORY</u>:
   Weakness or loss of sensation in any extremity; pain in the neck
   or back; difficulty moving back or spine; blood in urine or inability to void.

   <u>PHYSICAL EXAMINATION</u>:
   BEFORE MOVING THE PATIENT
   <u>Neck and back</u>: tenderness; normal alignment. Check for punch
      tenderness over the flanks.
   <u>Abdomen</u>: check for bladder distention.
   <u>Neurological</u>: check sensation movement and reflexes in all
      extremities.

NECK OR BACK TRAUMA
(Continued)

DIAGNOSTIC CONSIDERATIONS	HISTORY	PHYSICAL EXAM
Spine fracture (spinal cord injury may follow)	Neck or back pain.	Spinal tenderness or deformity.
Spinal cord injury or compression	Paralysis, numbness, inability to void.	Decreased sensation, muscle strength or reflexes (initially) are frequently noted; bladder distention may be observed.
Urinary tract trauma	Back or flank pain. Blood in urine.	May be normal or reveal punch tenderness over the flanks.

HISTORY

Descriptors:

General Descriptors: refer to inside cover.
Onset: when did the patient become aware of a tremor.
Location: is the tremor symmetrical.
Aggravating factors: does the tremor occur at rest or only
  on movement; what is the effect of anxiety and alcohol.

Associated Symptoms:
Anxiety or depression; strange feelings (specify); seizures;
abnormal strength or sensation; disequilibrium; change in
writing; jaundice.

Medical History:
Alcoholism; delirium tremens; emotional problems; liver
disease; neurological disease; Parkinson's disease;
thyroid disease; drug addiction; syphilis.

Medications:
Alcohol; diphenylhydantoin (Dilantin); L-dopa; benztropine
(Cogentin); tranquilizers.

Family History:
Tremor; neurological disease.

PHYSICAL EXAMINATION

Measure: resting pulse; temperature.
Neck: thyroid enlargement.
Abdomen: ascites; enlarged liver or spleen.
Extremities: check for cogwheel rigidity.
Neurological: is tremor at rest, while maintaining posture or
  on finger-to-nose test only. Carefully observe gait,
  spontaneity of gestures, facial expression. Deep tendon
  reflexes.

DIAGNOSTIC CONSIDERATIONS	HISTORY	PHYSICAL EXAM

ACTION TREMOR (fine tremor present throughout movement of an extremity or while maintaining a position)

Anxiety	History of acute or chronic emotional stress.	Sweaty palms; tachycardia.
Drug withdrawl	Often a history of drug abuse, particularly alcohol.	Fever; tachycardia; delirious disorientation; occasionally liver or spleen enlargement; hyperactive reflexes.
Inherited	Family history of tremor; a tremor noted later in life, often relieved by alcohol.	
Hyperthyroidism	Weight loss despite good appetite; heat intolerance.	Enlarged thyroid; tachycardia; abnormally rapid relaxation phase of deep tendon reflexes.

PARKINSONIAN TREMOR (present at rest, often disappearing with movement)

	Deterioration of fine and gross motor skills.	Shuffling (festinating gait) and cogwheel rigidity of extremities; immobile facies.

INTENTION TREMOR (no tremor at rest; tremor increased when precise movement is attempted -- particularly on finger-to-nose testing)

	Often a past history of neurological disease; motor or sensory deficits may be associated.	Ataxic, unsteady gait; incoordination with complex acts.

Reference: Harrison's Principles of Internal Medicine. Seventh Edition. Pages 85-94.

HISTORY

Descriptors:

General descriptors: refer to inside cover.
Location: what part of the body was involved.
Past treatment or evaluation: when and how diagnosed; when and
  how treated; most recent chest xray, sputum exam, or TB skin
  test.

Associated Symptoms:

Fever; chills; night sweats; cough, hemoptysis; weight loss;
decreased appetite.

Medical History:

Alcoholism; chronic lung disease; diabetes.

Medications:

Isoniazid; ethambutal; streptomycin; para-aminosalicylic acid;
rifampin; adrenal steroids.

Family History:

Tuberculosis.

Environmental History:

Have chest xray and skin test been performed on persons in
close contact with the patient prior to treatment. Try to
identify the person who might have transmitted tuberculosis
to the patient. Is the patient a smoker; has he worked with
rock dust or in a foundry.

PHYSICAL EXAMINATION

Measure: temperature; weight.
Chest: rales.

GENERAL CONSIDERATIONS

Active pulmonary tuberculosis may be associated with chronic
cough, night sweats and weight loss.

Persons who are at a high risk for developing active tuberculosis are:
1) Household contacts of persons with active pulmonary
   tuberculosis.
2) Persons who have had a recent change in their tuberculin
   status from negative to positive.

GENERAL CONSIDERATIONS

3) Persons who have had tuberculosis which was not adequately treated.
4) Persons with positive tuberculin skin tests who are also very old, very young, or suffering from concurrent disease (diabetes mellitus, silicosis, after gastrectomy, lymphoma, Hodgkin's disease). Persons with positive tuberculin skin tests who are receiving immunosuppressive therapy or chronic steroid medication are also at increased risk of developing active tuberculosis.
5) Persons with a positive tuberculin skin test having a chest xray which demonstrated evidence of non-progressive pulmonary tuberculosis.

Primary considerations in approaching the patient with known tuberculosis are:
1) How was the tuberculosis diagnosed.
2) What treatment was given. How long was it given.
3) What type of medical followup has been provided for the patient.
4) Were the contacts of the person with tuberculosis given a tuberculin skin test and diagnostic chest xrays.

Reference: Harrison's Principles of Internal Medicine.
Seventh Edition. Pages 858 - 870.

HISTORY

Descriptors:

General descriptors: refer to inside cover.
Onset: when was twitching first noted; what area (s) of the body are involved.
Aggravating factors: does twitching occur principally when falling asleep, following fatigue, or with anxiety.
Past treatment or evaluation: past neurological or electromyogram examinations, if any.

Associated Symptoms:
Muscle weakness; recent joint pains, or fever; skin rash; convulsions.

Medical History:
Rheumatic fever; neurological disease; birth injury; mental retardation; emotional disease.

Medications:
Phenothiazines (Thorazine).

Family History:
Dementia or similar "twitches".

Environmental History:
Twitching rarely follows use of insecticides.

PHYSICAL EXAMINATION

General: examine area of "twitching"; can the patient voluntarily suppress the abnormal movement.
Neurological: check muscles for strength and evidence of muscle atrophy; deep tendon reflexes; plantar reflex.

If age less than 16:
Heart: murmurs.

GENERAL CONSIDERATIONS

Tremors are rhythmic involuntary movements of the extremities (see TREMOR) whereas twitches are sudden jerking movements of part of the body that are usually not rhythmic.

GENERAL CONSIDERATIONS

Types of twitching movements are listed below.

Tics: Rapid repetitive movements which are most marked during
periods of stress and can be voluntarily suppressed. Common
tics are blinking, sniffing, or contracting one side of the
face.

Myoclonus: Very rapid, irregular asynchronous jerks which
may normally involve all extremities when one is falling
asleep. When myoclonic movements are not associated with
falling asleep or are persistent they are often associated
with convulsive disorders and neurological disease.

Chorea: Widespread rapid jerky movements which are usually
irregular and in variable locations. Choreiform movements
occuring in the child who has had a recent history of joint
pains and fever should be considered strong evidence of
rheumatic fever. Heart murmurs and a transient marginated
erythematous skin rash may also be noted.
   Persistent choreiform movements are associated with
chronic phenothiazine drug ingestion and neurological disorders (e.g. Huntington's chorea, cerebral palsy); other
neurological abnormalities or mental retardation may be
noted on examination.

Fasciculations: Brief irregular contractions of small
muscle units. These contractions may be so fine that
the muscle appears to shiver. Fasciculations are frequently observed in fatigued muscles. Persistent fasciculations associated with muscle weakness, hyperreflexia or
spasticity are usually secondary to degeneration of the
spinal cord (amyotrophic lateral sclerosis).

Reference: Harrison's Principles of Internal Medicine. Seventh
Edition. Pages 88 -91.

HISTORY

Descriptors:

General descriptors: refer to inside cover.
Onset: when and how first noted; how many times has the patient been bothered by ulcers since their onset.
Aggravating factors: anxiety; alcohol; aspirin; other food or medications.
Past treatment or evaluation: results of most recent upper gastrointestinal series or gastroscopy; previous treatment; previous diet.

Associated Symptoms:

Anxiety/depression; weight loss; weakness; abdominal pain; nausea; vomiting blood; tarry stools.

Medical History:

Gastric surgery; liver disease; arthritis; chronic lung disease; alcoholism.

Medications:

Aspirin; adrenal steroids (prednisone); warfarin (Coumadin); indomethacin (Indocin); alcohol; antacids; anticholinergics; sedatives; tranquilizers.

Family History:

Ulcer disease.

PHYSICAL EXAMINATION

Measure: Blood pressure, pulse – lying and standing.
Abdomen: tenderness, masses.
Rectal: stool for occult blood.

GENERAL CONSIDERATIONS

Peptic ulcer disease frequently recurs . To avoid recurrences and minimize serious consequences of active peptic ulcer disease the patient should be aware of:

1) Aggravating factors: caffein, cigarettes, alcohol, certain medications (aspirin, indomethacin, prednisone) and spicy foods.

2) The importance of strict adherence to a treatment regimen once symptoms occur.

3) The signs of gastrointestinal bleeding: melena, vomiting blood and orthostatic weakness.

Reference: Harrison's Principles of Internal Medicine. Seventh Edition. Pages 1431-1447.

HISTORY

Descriptors:

General descriptors: refer to inside cover.
Onset: how long has the ulcer been present.

Associated Symptoms:
Pain; muscle weakness or change in sensation; aching leg
muscles caused by walking and relieved by a short rest
(claudication); fever, chills, joint pain; discharge from
ulcer.

Medical History:
Diabetes; high blood pressure; cardiovascular disease;
blood disease; syphilis; neurological disease; varicose
veins; kidney disease; liver disease; local antibiotics.

Medications:
Local creams, salves; iodides; bromides; insulin; antihypertensives; digitalis; diuretics.

Environmental History:
Recurrent trauma to area.

PHYSICAL EXAMINATION

Measure: blood pressure; pulse; weight.
Extremities: elevate for 45 seconds and observe the location and degree of leg pallor. Hang the legs in a dependent position and note how long it takes for normal
color to return (usually 10 seconds) and for the cutaneous
veins of the feet to fill (usually 15 seconds).

Examine the ulcer. Note if the margin is red or blue,
hard or thickened. Is there surrounding erythema, brown
discoloration or edema. Are there varicose veins.
Nodes: check for enlargement of inguinal and popliteal
nodes.
Pulses: check pulses in legs.
Neurological: check vibration sense in legs.

GENERAL CONSIDERATIONS

Major concerns in the evaluation of leg ulcers are:
1) has edema been kept to a minimum, 2) are there symptoms

GENERAL CONSIDERATIONS

of cancer (persistent ulcer not responding to treatment
having hard thickened borders), 3) are there signs of infection (fever, local lymphadenopathy, spreading margin
of ulcer).

Arterial ulcers are often painful, have a red or blue
border and occur commonly on the feet. Claudication,
hypertension, diabetes and angina frequently coexist. Decreased pulses, poor venous filling time, blanching with
elevation, dependent redness of skin, and mild pitting
edema are often noted.

Ulcers associated with venous stasis and those associated
with chronic edema in the legs (severe heart failure, liver
disease or kidney disease) usually are found at or above
the ankle. Brown discoloration of the involved lower leg
and superficial venous varicosities are frequently noted.

Other causes of leg ulcers include reactions to iodide
and bromide medications and the result of poor pain sensation in the legs (syphilis, diabetes, or other neurological disease).

Reference: Harrison's Principles of Internal Medicine.
            Seventh Edition. Pages 267 - 278.

HISTORY

Descriptors:

General descriptors: refer to inside cover.
Who observed the patient and what were the events immediately prior to coma; what was the rate of change of consciousness.
Aggravating factors: trauma; if trauma, did the patient lose consciousness immediately; possible drug intoxication; alcoholism.

Associated Symptoms:
Fever; shaking chills; headache; sweating; tremulousness; convulsion; dyspnea; cough; nausea; vomiting; dysuria; dark urine; recent change in urinary output; change in sensation or motor function.

Medical History:
Any chronic disease; convulsive disorder; emotional problems; neurological disease; diabetes; hypertension; renal or liver disease; alcoholism; respiratory disease; cardiovascular disease.

Medications:
Any; in particular sedatives, tranquilizers, insulin, opiates.

False Positive:
The patient feigning "coma" may respond to a tickle of the lip or nasal vestibule; the eyelids often flutter.

PHYSICAL EXAMINATION

Measure: blood pressure; respiratory rate and pattern; pulse; temperature.
Mental status: is the patient drowsey or asleep; if asleep, is stimulation required to awaken him or does he remain unresponsive to any stimulation.

A COMPLETE PHYSICAL EXAMINATION IS REQUIRED. Note particularly:
Eyes: do eyes move in response to quick rotation of the head; do pupils respond to light; what is the resting position of the eyes and size of pupils.
Fundi: papilledema; hemorrhages.

PHYSICAL EXAMINATION
(Continued)

Neck: stiffness.
Chest: rales; wheezes; breath sounds.
Skin: cyanosis.
Extremities: edema; needle tracts.
Neurological: deep tendon reflexes; plantar reflex.

GENERAL CONSIDERATIONS

Before preceding with the evaluation of the comatose patient, the examiner must be sure that the patient has an adequate blood pressure and pulse and a satisfactory airway. Vital signs should be monitored throughout the evaluation.

The examiner should obtain a detailed history from anyone who may have been with the patient; frequently, this information leads directly to the diagnosis.

Structural brain damage (e.g. due to tumor, cerebrovascular disease or localized trauma) usually produces lateralizing neurological abnormalities (e.g. unequal pupils, unilateral paralysis or reflex changes).

When coma is due to diseases that affect the entire body (e.g. drug ingestion or a metabolic abnormality) the neurological changes are usually the same on both sides of the body.

Head injuries and drug or alcohol ingestion are the most common causes of stupor and coma.

Definitions:
Coma is only one aspect of a continuum of alternation of consciousness extending from drowsiness to death.

Confusion: refer to CONFUSION unless the patient is drowsy or stuporous.
Obtundation and stupor: patient is asleep but can be aroused by voice or gentle stimulation. The patient will return to sleep if stimulation is withheld.

GENERAL CONSIDERATIONS
 (Continued)

      Definitions:
       (Continued)

       Coma: the patient is totally unresponsive or unresponsive
          to all except very painful stimuli and returns to unrespon-
          siveness when these stimuli are withdrawn.

      CAUTION:
      Stupor and coma often cannot be fully evaluated on the basis
      of the history and physical examination alone. Laboratory
      tests and other methods of evaluation must be utilized fre-
      quently. Metabolic disorders, endocrine diseases, and unsus-
      pected intoxications are often not established as the cause
      of coma until specific laboratory analysis has been completed.

DIAGNOSTIC CONSIDERATIONS	HISTORY	PHYSICAL EXAM
TRANSIENT UNCONSCIOUSNESS: see BLACKOUT.		
CONVULSIONS: see CONVULSIONS.		
HEAD TRAUMA: see HEAD TRAUMA.		
POISONING OR DRUG OVERDOSE:		
Insulin overdose	Diabetic on insulin or oral hypogly-cemic agents; tremu-lousness, sweating and headache may precede the loss of consciousness.	Coma without lateralizing neurological signs.
Medications, poisons or alcohol	See OVERDOSE - POISONING.	

DIAGNOSTIC CONSIDERATIONS (Continued)	HISTORY	PHYSICAL EXAM
INFECTION:		
Meningitis/ Encephalitis	Headache; nausea; vomiting; fever; gradual lapse into coma.	Fever; stiff neck; occasionally papilledema and lateralizing neurological signs.
Secondary to severe systemic infection (pneumonia/ bacteremia)	Previous cough; dysuria; abdominal pain; fever or shaking chills before lapsing into coma.	Fever and hypotension may be present; no lateralizing neurological signs.
Brain abscess	Persistent headache; occasional fever.	Focal neurological abnormalities; papilledema or absence of venous pulsations; occasionally fever and stiff neck; localized pain while percussing cranium may be present.

METABOLIC AND ENDOCRINE: (usually no lateralizing neurological signs)

Diabetic ketoacidosis	Diabetic patient with recent fever, vomiting or surgical trauma; polyuria is often noted; gradual lapse into coma.	Hyperventilation with sweet smelling (ketone) breath; hypotension and decreased skin turgor are frequently present.
Respiratory failure	Usually a history of chronic lung disease and a recent respiratory infection gradually progressing to coma.	Shallow or slow respirations; decreased breath sounds and poor respiratory chest wall movement; rales, wheezes and cyanosis may be present.
Chronic renal failure	History of chronic renal disease; gradual lapse into coma.	Pallor is usually apparent.

DIAGNOSTIC CONSIDERATIONS	HISTORY	PHYSICAL EXAM

METABOLIC AND ENDOCRINE: (usually no lateralizing neurological signs). (Continued)

Acute renal failure	Decreased urine output; hematuria; nausea; one week later dyspnea, drowsiness are noted.	Rales; hypertension and peripheral edema may be present.

OTHER metabolic and endocrine causes of coma not listed above include: hypernatremia; hyponatremia; hypercalcemia; metabolic acidosis; renal or hepatic failure; hyper- and hypothyroidism; hyperthermia (heat stroke); adrenal or pituitary failure.

CEREBROVASCULAR DISEASE:

Intracranial hemorrhage	Sudden severe headache, nausea and vomiting with rapid loss of consciousness.	Fever; stiff neck; hypertension; lateralizing neurological signs; subhyaloid hemorrhages and papilledema are often present.
Hypertensive encephalopathy	Often a history of previous hypertension; encephalopathy may occur in the third trimester of pregnancy (eclampsia).	Diastolic blood pressure usually more than 140 mm of mercury; papilledema and retinal hemorrhages are common; lateralizing neurological signs may be present.
Cerebral infarction	Older patients previous "stroke", heart attack, chronic hypertension or diabetes increase the probability of the patient having cerebral infarction; patient may have suffered small reversible neurological deficits prior to the loss of consciousness; rapid	Lateralizing neurological signs are usually present.

DIAGNOSTIC CONSIDERATIONS	HISTORY	PHYSICAL EXAM
CEREBROVASCULAR DISEASE:		
Cerebral infarction (continued)	onset of symptoms suggest embolism of a cerebral vessel; slow, stepwise development of symptoms suggests thrombosis of a cerebral vessel.	See preceding page.
BRAIN TUMOR:	Chronic persistent headache progressing to nausea, vomiting and coma; gradual development of neurological deficits.	Lateralizing neurological signs; papilledema often present; retinal venous pulsations are often absent.
SHOCK:	Recent history of infection or bleeding may be obtained.	No lateralizing neurological signs; hypotension; cold, clammy skin.
FEIGNED COMA:	Often a history of emotional problems is obtained.	Vital signs and neurological examination are normal; eyelids often flutter; tickling of the nasal vestibule and lips often causes the patient to move.

<u>Reference</u>: Harrison's Principles of Internal Medicine. Seventh Edition. Pages 116-125.

HISTORY

Descriptors:

General descriptors: refer to inside cover.

Associated Symptoms:
Sore throat or pain on swallowing; pain in face or teeth;
runny nose; pain in ears; ringing or decreased hearing in
ears; cough; chest pain; sputum production; trouble breathing; muffled speaking; drooling.

Medical History:
Any history of illness or allergies.

Medications:
Any, especially recent antibiotics.

Environmental History:
Contact with someone with a streptococcal infection.

PHYSICAL EXAMINATION

Measure: temperature; respiratory rate.
Ear: check external canal and tympanic membrane.
Nose: discharge, polyps.
Sinus: tenderness.
Throat: redness; exudate; asymetry of tonsils; (Do not use
   instrument in children with drooling and severe stridor).
Neck: lymphadenopathy.
Lungs: localized rales or wheezes.

GENERAL CONSIDERATIONS

The viral upper respiratory infection (URI) is probably
the commonest cause of self-limited illness.

The adult with viral URI usually has only mild fever and
usually feels better within several days without therapy unless he has superimposed streptococcal pharyngitis, pneumonia
or mononucleosis. The child with viral URI, on the other
hand, may experience high fever.

The major considerations are to be sure that the patient
with the URI type syndrome does not have streptococcal
pharyngitis, otitis media or bacterial pneumonia. Rare but
serious complications are epiglottitis and pharyngeal abscess.

DIAGNOSTIC CONSIDERATIONS	HISTORY	PHYSICAL EXAM
Viral "URI" (common cold)	Runny nose; lethargy, mild headache; cough; often sore throat.	Swollen nasal mucous membranes; fever (mild in adults).
Pharyngitis (streptococcal or viral)	Sore throat; history of contact with strep-tococcal infection in-creases risk for streptococcal pharyn-gitis.	Abnormal throat exam. Lymphadenopathy and fever are more often present in strepto-coccal pharyngitis.
Sinusitis	Nasal discharge; facial pain.	Sinus tenderness.
Allergic rhinitis	Chronic or seasonal runny nose, and sneez-ing. Often aggravated by dusts or pollens.	Nasal polyps or nasal discharge are often noted.
Ear infection	Ear pain.	Abnormal ear exam. Fever (in children).
Mononucleosis	Sore throat; lethargy.	Fever. Posterior cer-vical lymphadenopathy and splenomegaly is usually present. Ab-normal throat exam.
Pneumonia	Cough; fever; chills; increased amount of green or yellow sputum; pleuritic chest pain.	Fever; localized rales or wheezes on lung exam.
Peritonsillar abscess	Severe throat pain.	Fever; often unilateral swollen tonsil which may obliterate the nor-mal architecture of the pharynx.
Epiglottitis	Extremely painful swallowing and con-sequent heavy drool-ing; difficulty breathing; muffled speech.	Fever; drooling; stridor cherry red swollen epi-glottis (if epiglottitis is suspected don't look in pharynx).

HISTORY

Descriptors:

General descriptors: refer to inside cover.
Onset: has patient been able to void in the last 12 hours.
Location: is there flank pain.
Radiation: does flank pain radiate to groin.
Past treatment or evaluation: When was the last urinalysis or
    kidney X-ray (IVP).

Associated Symptoms:
Low back or abdominal pain; passing stone or gravel; fever
or chills; pain on urination or frequent urination; urgency to
void; dark or bloody urine; decreased force of urine stream;
urination at night; uncontrolled urine; recent perineal or
abdominal trauma.

Medical History:
Kidney stones; recurrent urinary tract infections; kidney,
bladder or prostate disease; diabetes; neurological disease;
high blood pressure.

Medications:
Antibiotics; any others.

PHYSICAL EXAMINATION

Measure: temperature; blood pressure.
Abdomen: masses, tenderness; punch tenderness of flanks;
    attempt to percuss bladder.
Rectal (male): prostate tenderness or enlargement.
Extremities: edema.

            If dribbling of urine, uncontrolled urine
            or frequent urinary tract infection, check:

Genital-Rectal: do pelvic exam. Check for cystocoele, urethro-
    coele.
Extremities: reflexes in lower legs; plantar reflex.
Neurological: Perineal sensation.

DIAGNOSTIC CONSIDERATIONS	HISTORY	PHYSICAL EXAM
Dark Urine or Blood in Urine	See DARK URINE	
Excessive Urination (increase in total volume)	See EXCESSIVE DRINKING-EXCESSIVE URINATION	

DIAGNOSTIC CONSIDERATIONS	HISTORY	PHYSICAL EXAM
Painful Urination		
Associated with urethral discharge	Males with no history of gonorrhea contacts are usually suffering from "nonspecific urethritis".	Watery mild penile discharge.
	For other considerations see V.D. or DISCHARGE, VAGINA.	
Cystitis	Painful urination, urgency to void and frequent urination; fever and chills. Blood in urine is occasionally noted. May be asymptomatic or present only with fever and irritability in the child.	Fever.
Pylonephritis	Painful urination, frequent urination, flank pain. Fever and chills may be more frequent and severe in diabetic patients. May be asymptomatic or present only with fever and irritability in the child.	Fever; punch tenderness of flanks.
Kidney stone	History of blood in urine or passing "gravel". Severe flank or abdominal pain ("colic") radiating to groin or testicle.	Flank tenderness is usually noted.

DIAGNOSTIC CONSIDERATIONS	HISTORY	PHYSICAL EXAM
Inability to Void; Hesitancy, Decreased Force of Urine Stream		
Acute urinary retention	Unable to void. Lower abdominal discomfort. May have a history of prostate trouble or renal stones. May have recently taken anticholinergic medications.	Bladder can usually be palpated or percussed on abdominal examination.
Urethral obstruction (usually due to prostatic hypertrophy)	Older male. Difficulty initiating voiding; frequency, dribbling, nocturia also noted. Decreased force of urine stream.	Prostate is often enlarged but may be normal in size.
Uncontrolled Urination		
Stress incontinence	Usually females following multiple pregnancies. Incontinence occurs on laughing, coughing, straining.	Cystocoele or urethrocoele may be seen on pelvic examination.
Incontinence due to neurological problem	Patient may have low back pain, a history of diabetes, or other neurological disease (stroke, dementia). Lower extremities may be weak, painful or numb.	Decreased perineal sensation and hyperactive deep tendon reflexes or Babinski response may be noted in the legs.
Frequent Urination at Night (Nocturia)		
Following fluid, alcohol or coffee intake before bed	History of ingestion of these substances with resultant diuresis at night.	Normal.

DIAGNOSTIC CONSIDERATIONS	HISTORY	PHYSICAL EXAM

Frequent Urina-tion at Night
(Continued)

| Secondary to fluid reten-tion states | Patient may note short-ness of breath or edema of the legs. Common in congestive heart failure. | May reveal rales in lungs or peripheral edema. |
| Secondary to urethral obstruction | See discussion of urethral obstruction above. | |

Reference: Harrison's Principles of Internal Medicine. 7th edition, Pages 237-246.

HISTORY

Descriptors:

General descriptors: refer to inside cover.
During bleeding, how many pads per day. Date of last menstrual period. Timing of bleeding in relation to menses.
Aggravating factors: possibility of pregnancy. (if probable pregnancy and bleeding, see ABORTION)
Past treatment or evaluation: thyroid tests; last pap test or pelvic exam.

Associated Symptoms:

Emotional stress; anxiety; depression; hot flashes; change in weight; heat intolerance; change in hair distribution or texture; breast engorgement; nausea, vomiting, abdominal pain; fever, chills; bruising, passing "tissue" (if bleeding).

Medical History:

Pelvic inflammatory disease; diabetes; thyroid disease; drug addiction; emotional disease; pregnancies, miscarriages, abortions; onset of pubic and axcillary hair growth, breast development, and periods.

Medications:

Birth control pills; intra-uterine device; warfarin (Coumadin); thyroid pills; adrenal steroids.

Family History:

Age of onset and cessation of menses in female parent or sibling; bleeding problems.

PHYSICAL EXAMINATION

Measure: blood pressure; pulse; temperature.
Genital: pelvic exam: check carefully for masses or tenderness. Perform pap test.
Skin: Secondary sex characteristics: pubic-axillary hair (quantity, distribution); breast development.

GENERAL CONSIDERATIONS:

The first distinction to make is between the various menstrual abnormalities: amenorrhea (no vaginal bleeding), dysmenorrhea (painful menses) and abnormal bleeding (too much and/or irregular bleeding).

Amenorrhea: Primary amenorrhea (never had menses) is usually due to delayed puberty, but may reflect a systemic disease (tuberculosis, diabetes, anorexia nervosa), thyroid disease or a congenital problem (gonadal dysgenesis, hypoplastic uterus).

<u>GENERAL CONSIDERATIONS</u>: (Continued)

Puberty may normally start as late as 16 years.

Secondary amenorrhea is most frequently a sign of pregnancy
(see PREGNANT), but may also be due to a large number of other
causes (pituitary insufficiency, ovarian and other endocrine
disorders, and some systemic diseases).

<u>Dysmenorrhea</u> is a common problem, particularly during adoles-
cence and is usually not associated with any serious disorder.
However, it may have a symptom of endometriosis or pelvic
inflammatory disease. (see CRAMPS, MENSTRUAL)

<u>Abnormal Menstrual Bleeding</u> is common near the start (menarche)
and the end (menopause) of the reproductive years, when it may
be a "normal" finding. It may also be a manifestation of
problems in an early pregnancy (see ABORTION) or of benign or
malignant tumors of the cervix or uterus. In addition, it may
accompany a large number of other disorders including those of
an endocrine, ovarian, metabolic, infectious or emotional
nature.

<u>Reference</u>: Harrison's Principles of Internal Medicine. 7th edition,
             Pages 246-247.

HISTORY:

Descriptors:
General descriptors: refer to inside cover.
Why does patient suspect he has venereal disease; does patient
have many sexual contacts; do any of the sexual contacts have
VD; are any sexual contacts promiscuous.
Character: color of penile or vaginal discharge.
Past treatment and evaluation: past blood tests for syphilis.
Past treatment or evaluation for gonorrhea.

Associated Symptoms: swollen lymph nodes; dysuria; genital sores;
pelvic pain; fever or chills; conjunctivitis; joint pains; recent skin rash.

Medical History: syphilis; gonorrhea; pelvic inflammatory disease;
allergy to penicillin or ampicillin.

Environmental: nature of sexual exposure--oral, anal or genital.

PHYSICAL EXAMINATION:

Genital:
Female: pelvic exam with culture of cervix.
Male: examine urethral discharge. If no discharge perform rectal
examination and massage prostate to obtain a discharge.

GENERAL CONSIDERATIONS:

Syphilis and gonorrhea are frequently present simultaneously.
Syphilis should be considered in the differential diagnosis of
any lesion of the external genitalia. Fear of contacting venereal
disease may be a more common concern to the patient than the actual
presence of signs or symptoms of disease because gonorrhea is frequently asymptomatic in the male and female.

Not all vaginal or uretheral discharges are due to VD. (See DISCHARGE,
VAGINA and the nonvenereal diagnostic considerations for the male
listed on the following pages).

DIAGNOSTIC CONSIDERATIONS	HISTORY	PHYSICAL EXAM
Syphilis	Painless genital ulcer may be noted during first 6 weeks after exposure. Generalized rash may follow.	Very firm nontender ulcer; enlarged lymph nodes may be noted. Later a generalized papulosquamous rash with lymph node enlargement is frequently observed in untreated cases.
Chancroid	Painful genital ulcer; inguinal swelling.	Superficial, soft tender ulcer with ragged undermined edges and yellow exudate; tender enlarged lymph nodes may be noted.
Herpes virus	Often watery discharge and painful urination are noted; painful genital lesions.	Multiple vesicles on penis or on labial inner surface; occasional inguinal adenopathy.
Granuloma inguinale or Lymphogranuloma venereum	Tender lymph nodes and progressive ulceration of inguinal region often occurs.	Marked perineal inflammation and skin destruction is often noted.
Trichomonas urethritis	Urethral itching; mild dysuria and thick, clear penile discharge; sexual partners often reinfect one another. In female: usually severe vaginal pruritus and discharge. Odor is often present.	Thick clear penile discharge. In female: vaginal mucosa inflamed; discharge is frothy, gray, green or yellow.

NON-VENEREAL CAUSES OF PENILE DISCHARGE:
(Continued)

DIAGNOSTIC CONSIDERATIONS	HISTORY	PHYSICAL EXAM

NON-VENEREAL CAUSES OF VAGINAL DISCHARGE: See DISCHARGE, VAGINA

NON-VENEREAL CAUSES OF PENILE DISCHARGE:

DIAGNOSTIC CONSIDERATIONS	HISTORY	PHYSICAL EXAM
Non-specific urethritis	Minimal clear penile discharge with mild dysuria.	Clear watery penile discharge.
Reiters syndrome	Dysuria; frequent and persistent, thick penile discharge; the patient is usually a young male who also complains of migratory joint pains and conjunctivitis.	Persistent, thick, green yellow penile discharge. Gram stain does not reveal gonoccocus.

HISTORY

Descriptors:
> General descriptors: refer to inside cover.
> Onset: how much vomiting or wretching before blood noticed;
>   total amount of blood; previous attacks.
> Character: bright red blood in vomit or "coffee ground"
>   material.
> Past treatment or evaluation: results of upper gastrointestinal
>   series; esophagoscopy or gastroscopy; previous requirement
>   for transfusions.

Associated Symptoms:
> Weakness; feeling faint when standing; skin bruising; red
> spots on skin; abdominal distention; abdominal pain; black
> tarry or bloody bowel movements; jaundice.

Medical History:
> Esophageal varices; ulcer disease; gastritis; liver disease;
> alcoholism; blood disease; bleeding disorder; previous gastro-
> intestinal bleeding.

Medications:
> Aspirin; warfarin (Coumadin); indomethacin (Indocin); alcohol;
> adrenal steroids.

Family History:
> Bleeding disorder.

False positive:
> Bleeding from nose or mouth and coughing up blood may be re-
> ported as vomiting blood.

PHYSICAL EXAMINATION

> Measure: blood pressure and pulse lying and sitting .
> Mental status: memory; proverbs; ability to calculate.
> Throat: mouth - telangiectasia.
> Abdomen: ascites, liver and spleen size.
> Rectal: examination with stool for occult blood.
> Skin: spider angiomata, ecchymosis, petechiae, jaundice,
>   pallor.

DIAGNOSTIC CONSIDERATIONS	HISTORY	PHYSICAL EXAM
Peptic ulcer	Epigastric pain often relieved by food or antacids; aggravated by aspirin, adrenal steroids, alcohol; black or tarry bowel movements.	Melena; epigastric tenderness.
Gastritis	Often painless; usually secondary to excessive aspirin or alcohol ingestion.	Melena; minimal abdominal tenderness.
Esophageal varices	Most often seen in chronic alcoholics with cirrhosis of the liver.	Spider angiomata; ascites; splenomegaly; jaundice; melena; abnormal mental status exam may also be present.
Esophageal tear	Often a history of prolonged wretching preceding bloody vomitus.	Often normal.
Bleeding disorders	May have a family history of bleeding or a history or bleeding easily and excessively.	Petechiae, telangiectasias and ecchymoses may be noted on the skin or mucous membranes.

PEDIATRIC CONSIDERATIONS

Vomiting of blood is rare in children. The commonest cause is secondary to blood ingestion from bleeding in the nose and mouth, from the mother's bleeding nipple or from the bleeding of childbirth. Newborns occasionally develop hemorrhagic disease and bruise and bleed spontaneously at many sites.

Reference: Harrison's Principles of Internal Medicine. Seventh Edition. Pages 218-221.

HISTORY

Descriptors:

General descriptors: refer to inside cover.
Aggravating factors: is patient on diet; what exactly does
   patient eat.
Past treatment and evaluation: how much weight loss is documented during what period of time.

Associated Symptoms:

Change in appetite; anxiety; depression; loose stools; heat
intolerance; nausea; vomiting; excessive urination; abdominal
pain.

Medications:

Any.

Environmental:

Any change in family, finances or job.

PHYSICAL EXAMINATION

Measure: weight; height.
Neck: check for thyroid enlargement.
Abdomen: masses; tenderness; liver size.
Rectal exam: test stool for occult blood.
Extremities: muscle wasting; edema; check skin turgor.
Neurological: reflexes; check for relaxation phase of
   deep tendon reflexes.

GENERAL CONSIDERATIONS

The range of normal daily caloric intake for a moderately
active adult is 2200-2800 calories for men and 1800-2100 for
women who are not pregnant or lactating.

Weight loss usually results from inadequate caloric intake
(see ANOREXIA if patient complains of decreased appetite).
Weight loss in the face of adequate caloric intake may occur
when:

   a. the body wastes calories (uncontrolled diabetes;
      intestinal malabsorption).
   b. there are excessive caloric requirements (increased
      physical activity, pregnancy, hyperthyroidism,
      chronic infections or malignancy).

Reference: Harrison's Principles of Internal Medicine. Seventh
   Edition. Pages 230-231.

HISTORY

Expected Developmental Milestones	Average age	Range
Lifts head when prone		0-4 weeks
Smiles responsively	1 month	0-8 weeks
Vocalizes	6 weeks	2-10 weeks
Rolls over; follows 180 degrees	3 months	2-4 months
Turns head to sound	3½ months	3-5 months
Reaches for objects	4 months	3-5 months
Transfers objects; sits without support	6 months	5-8 months
Imitates sounds	7 months	5-9 months
Pulls self to stand; crawls	8 months	6-11 months
Pincer grasp; "Mama", "Dada" specifically; stands well alone	11 months	9-15 months
Walks well	13 months	7-16 months
3 words other than "Mama", "Dada"	13 months	11-21 months
Walks up steps	17 months	13-23 months
Knows one body part	19 months	13-23 months
Uses plurals; 2-4 word sentences	19 months	15-23 months

Environmental:
1) Attitudes and anxieties of parents.
2) Diet; fluoride content of water source.
3) Safety precautions (seat belts; accessibility of medications, household cleansers and other chemicals). Is IPECAC available at home.
4) Sleeping arrangements and general sanitary facilities for the child.

PHYSICAL EXAMINATION (and expected findings)

Measure (every visit):
Weight: birth weight doubles in first 6 months; triples in first year; quadruples by end of second year.
Length: increases by ¼ birth length in first year.
Head: circumference. (Compare to standard charts).

Head: fontanel (anterior) normally closes between 10-14 months.
Eyes: mild strabismus disappears by 6 months; should follow objects by 4 months. Funduscopic--look for red reflex. (See also screening for amblyopia--EYE PROBLEMS).

PHYSICAL EXAMINATION
(Continued)

Mouth: teeth appear at the sixth month to 1 year.

Chest: respiratory rate 30 in first year; 25 second year and 20 by the eighth year.

Cardiac: 130 beats at birth; 105 beats in second year and 80 beats by third year. Blood pressure should be checked at least by the fourth year (when it is normally 85/60).

Abdomen: small umbilical hernias are common in the first year; palpate carefully for any masses.

Genitals: Male: testes descend by 1 year in almost all cases; hydrocoeles are common in the first year.
   Female: check for appearance of genitalia.

Extremities: Feet: often retain an in utero position but have unrestricted full range of motion. Persistent toe-in deformities or feet with decreased range of motion require correction.
   Hips: hip range of motion should be done every visit on young females. Check carefully for clicks or disparity of range of motion in hips.

Neurological: plantar extensor reflex normal up to 2 years; suck and grasp reflexes normally disappear by 4 months.

GENERAL CONSIDERATIONS

At no other period in life are changes occuring faster than they are in the young infant. The purpose of the well baby check is to make certain that both the child's physical development and the environmental inputs afforded the child are adequate to allow appropriate social, mental and physical maturation.

Parents are also experiencing a significant change in their lives and opportunity should be provided for them to talk of their feelings.

Sensory, social and motor milestones must be scrupulously observed as indicators of the proper maturing of the infant. Examiners should constantly remind themselves of the purpose of the well baby check and avoid restricting themselves to physical and gross motor assessment alone.

WELL BABY CHECK
(Continued)

GENERAL CONSIDERATIONS
(Continued)

Usual Immunization schedule:

2 months	Diptheria, tetanus, pertussis, and trivalent oral polio virus vacine.
4 months	Diptheria, tetanus, pertussis, and trivalent oral polio virus vacine.
6 months	Diptheria, tetanus, pertussis, and trivalent oral polio virus vacine.
9 months	Tuberculin skin test.
1 year	Measles, (tuberculin).
1-12 years	Rubella, mumps.
1½ years	Diptheria, tetanus, pertussis, and trivalent oral polio virus vacine.
4-6 years	Diptheria, tetanus, pertussis, and trivalent oral polio virus vacine.
14-16 years	Tetaus and diptheria toxoids and thereafter every ten years barring intercurrent contaminated wounds.

Included below are <u>simple</u> definitions of words used in the HISTORY section of the Data Base Pages.

ABRASION - superficial scraping of skin.

ABSCESS - a localized collection of pus.

ACUTE - sudden; having a short course.

ADRENAL - a gland near the kidney that is important in the body's reaction to stress.

AMBLYOPIA - a disease in which a 'lazy' eye does not fix accurately on objects; may eventually cause squint (cross eyes, wall eyes) and blindness of the 'lazy' eye.

ANALGESIA - absence (or decrease) of pain sensation.

ANEMIA - deficiency of blood quantity or quality.

ANGINA - a pattern of chest pain usually due to disease of the heart's arteries.

ANKYLOSING SPONDYLITIS - a disease of young men causing persistent back pain and eventually resulting in fixation of the spine.

ANOREXIA - loss of appetite.

ANOREXIA NERVOSA - a disease in which the patient will not eat and may die of starvation.

ANTIARRYTHMICS - medications used to regulate the abnormal beating of the heart.

ANTIBIOTICS - medications used to help the body fight bacterial or fungus infections.

ANTIBODY - a blood protein (globulin) useful in helping the body fight infections.

ANTICHOLINERGICS - medications which block nerves that help activate digestive processes.

ANTICONVULSANTS - medications used to control convulsive (seizure) disorders.

ANTISPASMODICS - see Anticholinergics above.

APHASIA - loss of the ability to speak or write due to damage of the brain.

ARRHYTHMIA - abnormal beat of the heart.

ARTERIOGRAM - an x-ray study of dye injected into vessels carrying blood away from the heart.

ARTHRALGIA - joint aches causing no joint tenderness or destruction.

ASCITES - an abnormal collection of fluid in the abdomen (peritoneal cavity).

ASYMPTOMATIC - referring to a disease causing no patient complaints.

ATAXIA - unsteadiness; incoordination.

ATHEROSCLEROSIS - "hardening" of the arteries.

ATOPIC ECZEMA - see SKIN PROBLEMS Data Base Pages.

ATRIAL - pertaining to the two upper chambers of the heart which receive blood from the body and lungs.

AUTONOMIC - the involuntary part of the nervous system which controls bodily functions such as digestion or blood pressure.

AXILLARY - armpit.

BARIUM ENEMA - x-ray of the large bowel.

BILIARY - the drainage system of the liver (bile ducts, gall bladder).

BIOPSY - surgical removal of tissue for examination.

BIRTH TRAUMA - injury to the infant during birth.

BRONCHIECTASIS - chronic dilitations in the air passage ways to the lungs.

BRONCHODILATORS - medications which can dilate the air passages in the lung.

BURSITIS - inflammation of the lubricating sac near a joint.

CARDIOVASCULAR - pertaining to the heart and blood vessels.

CATHETER - a tube for withdrawing fluids from, or putting fluids into, the body.

CEREBROVASCULAR - pertaining to the blood vessels directly supplying the brain.

CHOLESTEROL and TRIGLYCERIDES - fatlike substances in the blood.

CHRONIC - not acute - of long duration.

CIRRHOSIS - scarring of the liver.

CLAUDICATION - calf pain caused by inadequate blood supply (see JOINT - EXTREMITY PAINS Data Base Pages).

COLIC - see ABDOMINAL PAIN - PEDIATRIC Data Base Pages.

COLITIS - inflammatory disease of the large bowel.

COMA - unconsciousness.

CONGESTIVE HEART FAILURE - failure of heart function causing the body to retain fluid; fluid retention often causes edema of the legs, shortness of breath and abnormal sounds in the lungs (rales).

CONJUNCTIVITIS - inflammation of the membrane that lines the eyelids and overlies the 'whites' of the eyes.

CONTACT DERMATITIS - skin inflammation caused by touching certain substances.

CONNECTIVE TISSUE DISEASE - disease of the tissue that supports most structures of the body (e.g., connective tissue is found in joints, blood vessels, tendons, skin, and muscles).

COSTOVERTEBRAL ANGLE - see FLANK.

CYANOSIS - blue colored skin due to insufficient oxygen in the blood.

CYST - a sac containing fluid.

CYSTIC FIBROSIS - a hereditary chronic disease often causing greasy foul smelling diarrhea, recurrent lung infections and death.

DEFECATION - having a bowel movement.

DELIRIUM - a confused state due to underlying disease.

DELIRIUM TREMENS - delirium due to cessation of chronic alcohol ingestion.

DEMENTIA - usually irreversible mental deterioration.

DENTITION - referring to the teeth.

DERMATITIS - inflammation of the skin.

DESENSITIZATION - causing a person to no longer react to a substance.

DIAPHORESIS - profuse sweating.

DIGITALIS - a drug useful for strengthening the heart.

DIPLOPIA - double vision.

DISTAL - farthest from the body.

DISTENTION - being swollen or stretched.

DIURETICS - 'fluid' pills; medications which cause increased urine secretion.

DIVERTICULA - small blind pouches most often found extending from the wall of the large bowel or esophagus.

DYSGENESIS - defective development.

DYSFUNCTION - abnormal function.

DYSMENORRHEA - painful menstrual periods.

DYSPAREUNIA - painful sexual intercourse in women.

DYSPHAGIA - difficulty swallowing.

DYSPNEA - the sensation of being short of breath.

DYSURIA - painful urination.

ECCHYMOSES - bruises.

ECZEMA - see SKIN PROBLEMS Data Base Pages.

EDEMA - an abnormal increase in tissue fluid; edema is usually noted in the lungs or under the skin.

EMBOLUS - a blood clot that moves through the blood vessels.

EMPHYSEMA - a form of chronic lung disease.

ENCEPHALITIS - inflammation or infection of the brain.

ENDOCARDITIS - inflammation or infection of the heart.

ENDOMETRIOSIS - tissue from the uterus that collects in abnormal places.

ENURESIS - bed wetting.

ENTERITIS - inflammation of the small bowel.

EPIGLOTTITIS - inflammation of a structure in the throat which can block the air passages.

EPIGASTRIUM - the upper middle portion of the abdomen.

EPISTAXIS - nose bleed.

ERUCTATION - burping.

ERYTHEMA - redness.

EXCORIATION - scratching away of superficial skin.

EXOPHTHALMOS - bulging of the eyeballs.

EXPECTORATION - coughing up a substance.

EXUDATE - a fluid that often forms on injured surfaces and turns into a yellow crust when dry.

FECAL - pertaining to bowel movements.

FEMORAL - pertaining to structures on or near the thigh bone.

FIBRILLATION - fine spontaneous contraction of muscles.

FIBROCYSTIC - see Cystic Fibrosis.

FIBROID (LEIMYOMA) - a non-malignant muscular growth of the uterus.

FIBROSIS - scarring.

FISTULA - an abnormal passage; usually from the skin to an internal structure.

FLANK - the lateral back sides of the abdomen.

FLATULENCE - passing gas.

FOLATE - a vitamin.

GASTRIC - pertaining to the stomach.

GASTROENTERITIS - acute upset of bowel function.

GASTROINTESTINAL - pertaining to the stomach and bowels.

GASTROSCOPY - visualization of the stomach using a long tube.

GIDDY - light headed.

GLAUCOMA - abnormal high pressure in the eyeball.

GLOBULIN - a type of protein in the body.

GONOCOCCAL - pertaining to the bacteria causing gonorrhea.

GOUT - a disease causing acute painful joints in men.

GROSS - coarse or large.

HEAT STROKE - see HEAT STROKE Data Base Pages.

HEMATEMESIS - vomiting blood.

HEMATURIA - blood in urine.

HEMOPHILIA - a hereditary disease caused by a reduced ability of blood to form clots.

HEMOPTYSIS - coughing blood.

HEPATITIS - inflammation of the liver.

HEPATOMEGALY - large liver.

HEPATOSPLENOMEGALY - large liver and spleen.

HESITANCY - inability to begin urinating.

HIATUS HERNIA - an opening allowing the stomach to slide into the chest.

HIRSUTISM - abnormal hairiness.

HOT FLASHES - the sensation of fever associated with the menopause.

HYDROCEPHALUS - abnormal collection of fluid in the skull causing brain damage.

HYPERTENSION - abnormal elevation of blood pressure.

HYPERVENTILATION - prolonged rapid and deep breathing.

HYPOGLYCEMIA - low blood sugar.

HYPOPLASTIC - incompletely developed.

HYPOREFLEXIA - weak reflexes.

HYPOTENSION - abnormally low blood pressure.

INCONTINENCE - inability to control urine or bowel.

INFARCTION - death of tissue due to poor blood supply.

INFLAMMATION - the reaction of body tissues to injury characterized by swelling, warmth, tenderness and, when visible, redness.

INGUINAL - pertaining to the groin.

ISCHEMIA - a local or temporary lack of blood to tissue.

JAUNDICE - abnormal yellow skin or 'whites' of the eye (see JAUNDICE).

KETOACIDOSIS - a state when a person lacks sufficient substances
     in the blood (insulin) often resulting in coma, dehydration
     and abnormal acidification of the body fluids. Usually a
     problem of persons suffering from insulin-dependent diabetes.

LACERATION - a cut.

LACTATION - nursing; screting milk.

LESION - an abnormality (usually of the skin).

LETHARGY - strictly defined as drowsiness; often means "feeling
     tired out" (lassitude) in common usage.

LEUKOCYTE - white blood cell in body which helps fight infections.

LUMBAR PUNCTURE - placing a needle into the lower spine to with-
     draw fluid which surrounds the spinal cord.

LUPUS ERYTHEMATOSIS - a connective tissue disease.

LYMPH NODES - absorbent glandlike structures which collect
     drainage of a clear fluid from the body.

LYMPHADENOPATHY - enlargement of lymph nodes.

MALAISE - fatigue; generalized body discomfort.

MALIGNANCY - a disease tending to go from bad to worse. Usually
     a cancer.

MELENA - black tarry bowel movements.

MENIERE'S DISEASE - see DIZZINESS - VERTIGO Data Base Pages.

MENINGITIS - infection or inflammation of the covering of the brain.

MENORRHAGIA - heavy menstrual bleeding.

MENSES - menstrual periods.

MYALGIA - muscle aches.

MYELOGRAM - an x-ray study of dye injected around the spinal cord.

MYOCARDIAL INFARCTION - death of heart muscle due to an inadequate blood supply.

MYOGRAM - electrical measurement of muscle activity.

NASOGASTRIC INTUBATION - passing a tube from the nose to the stomach.

NECROSIS - death.

NEURODERMATITIS - nervous scratching.

NEUROLOGICAL - pertaining to the nervous system.

NEUROPATHY - disease of nerves.

NOCTURIA - having to urinate at night.

NODE - a lymph gland.

OBSTIPATION - severe constipation.

OBSTRUCTIVE PULMONARY DISEASE - a common form of chronic lung disease (emphysema).

ORCHITIS - inflammation of testicles.

ORTHOPNEA - inability to breath when lying down; relieved by sitting up.

ORTHOSTATIC - caused by standing up.

OSTEOARTHRITIS - the common arthritis of old age (degenerative arthritis).

OTITIS MEDIA - infection of the middle ear.

PALPITATION - sensation of heart beat.

PANCREATITIS - inflammation of the pancreas.

PARESTHESIA - an abnormal sensation (tingling, prickling, etc.).

PELVIC INFLAMMATORY DISEASE - usually gonorrhea.

PEPTIC ULCER - ulcer of the stomach duodenum or lower esophagus.

PERICARDIUM - the sac surrounding the heart.

PERINEAL - the area between the thighs.

PERIORAL - around the mouth.

PERIRECTAL - around the rectum.

PERITONEUM - the space between the bowels and the abdominal wall.

PETECHIAE - spot sized bleeding into the skin.

PHARYNGITIS - inflammation of the posterior throat.

PHENOTHIAZINES - medications that tend to sedate and control psychotic thoughts.

PHLEBITIS - inflammation of veins; blood clot is usually present.

PHOTOPHOBIA - abnormal intolerance of light.

PLEURISY - inflammation of the covering of the lungs. Usually painful.

PNEUMOTHORAX - an abnormal collection of air between the lungs and the chest wall.

POLYDIPSIA - excessive thirst (amount).

POLYP - a growth which protrudes into a cavity (e.g., nasal polyp, polyp of large bowel).

POLYPHAGIA - excessive appetite.

POLYURIA - excessive urination (amount).

POPLITEAL - the space behind the knee.

POSTPRANDIAL - after meals.

PRECORDIAL - region overlying the heart.

PRIMARY - first in order; principal.

PROCTOSCOPE - visualization of the lower bowel by passing a tube through the anus.

PRODOME - a symptom indicating the beginning of a disease.

PROLAPSE - falling out of position.

PRURITUS - itching.

PSORIASIS - see SKIN PROBLEMS Data Base Pages.

PULMONARY - pertaining to lungs.

PULSATILE - rhythmic movement.

PURULENT - containing pus.

PUSTULE - a small skin elevation filled with pus.

PYELOGRAM - an x-ray study of the kidneys after injecting dye
    into the blood.

RECTAL - the last portion of the large bowel.

RENAL - pertaining to kidneys.

RHEUMATIC FEVER - a disease, usually of children, with fever,
    joint pains and possible heart damage.

RHEUMATOID ARTHRITIS - a deforming chronic disease of joints.

RHINITIS - inflammation of the inside of the nose.

SCAPULA - shoulder blade.

SCLERAL ICTERUS - yellowing of the 'whites' of the eyes.

SECONDARY - second or inferior in order.

SECONDARY SEXUAL CHARACTERISTICS - sexual characteristics occurring
    at puberty that differentiate male from female (voice changes,
    muscle changes, breast changes, pubic, facial, axillary, and
    scalp hair changes, etc.).

SEIZURE - see CONVULSIONS Data Base Pages.

SIBLING - brother or sister.

SIGMOIDOSCOPE - see PROCTOSCOPE.

SIGN - any objective evidence of a disease.

SPUTUM - mucus coughed from the respiratory tract.

STENOSIS - narrowing.

STEROIDS - potent medications (with many side effects) that tend
   to reduce inflammation.

STRABISMUS - wall eyed, cross eyed.

STUPOR - see UNCONSCIOUS Data Base Pages.

SYMPTOM - a change in health which the person perceives and
   expresses.

SYNCOPE - temporary loss of consciousness.

SYNDROME - a set of symptoms which occur together.

SYSTEMIC - affecting the entire body.

TACHYCARDIA - excessively fast heart beat.

TENESMUS - urgency to have a bowel movement.

THROMBOPHLEBITIS - see PHLEBITIS.

TINNITUS - buzzing or ringing in the ears.

TOXEMIA - a dangerous hypertensive state of pregnant women.

TRAUMA - injury.

TURGOR - the consistency of the skin due to the fluid it contains.

URETHRA - the tube carrying urine from the bladder to the outside.

URTICARIA - hives.

VAGINITIS - inflammation of the vagina.

VALVULAR - pertaining to the valves of the heart.

VASCULAR - pertaining to blood vessels.